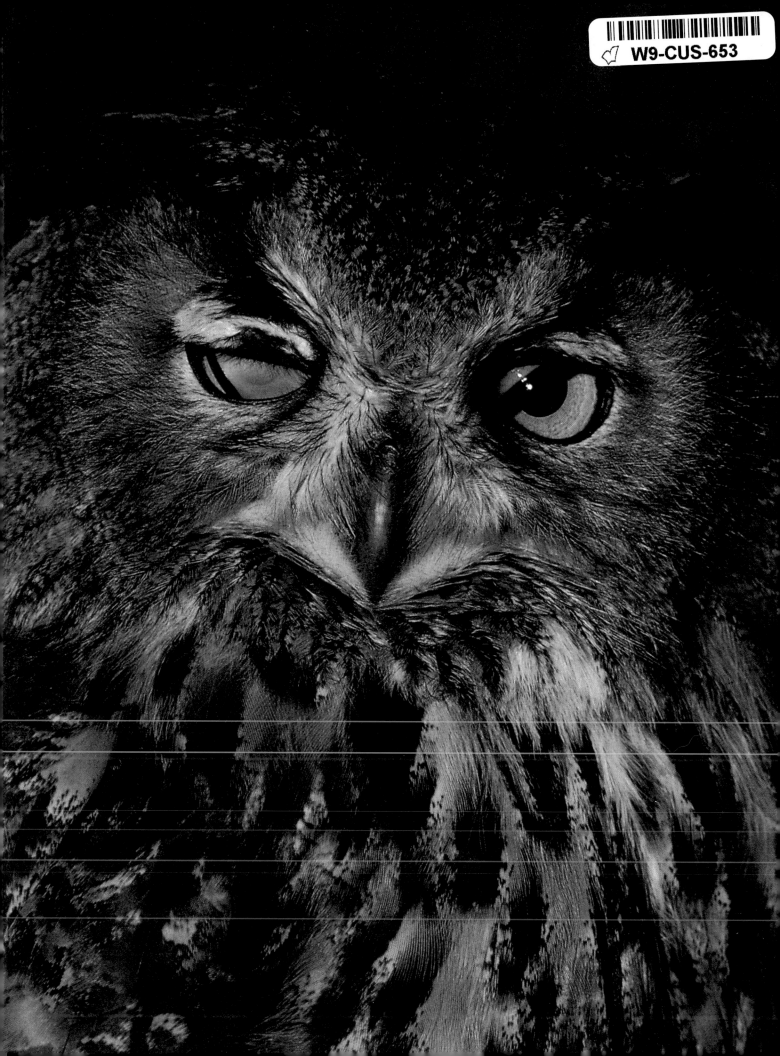

How Animals See

How Animals See

Other Visions of Our World

Sandra Sinclair

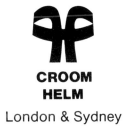

CROOM
HELM
London & Sydney

How
Animals
See

© 1985 Sandra Sinclair
This Edition published by Croom Helm Ltd, Provident House, Burrell
Row, Beckenham, Kent BR3 1AT, England

Croom Helm Australia Pty Ltd, First Floor, 139 King Street, Sydney,
NSW 2001, Australia

Sinclair, Sandra
  [Other visions of our world]. How animals see : other visions of our
  world
  1. Vision
  I. Title   II. How animals see : other visions of our world
  591.1'823   QP475

PRINTED IN BELGIUM
ISBN 0-7099-3336-3

To Essex, Taffy, Thai, Belle Gazoo,
Bimi, Duchess, and all the many
other creatures with whom I have
been fortunate enough to share my life.

Contents

Introduction XI

1. Forming an Image 1

2. Primitive Eyes 9

3. Spiders 14

4. Insects 21

5. Crustaceans 38

6. Cephalopods 43

7. Fish 49

8. Amphibians 69

9. Reptiles 75

10. Birds 88

11. Nocturnal Animals 101

12. Mammals 112

13. Primates 127

Bibliography 137

Index 143

Photo Credits 145

Foreword

When Sandra Sinclair started out on this project, she intended to produce a book that would give some possible insights about how a number of different animals might perceive the visual world. I suggested a few general textbook-type readings to her, along with a few articles from such journals as *Scientific American*. Sandra proved to be an avid student of the visual system, and it soon became clear that she would not be satisfied with a superficial treatment of the subject. We then started on a kind of one-to-one seminar in vision science that extended, before we knew it, over several years. My own research had been concentrated in a few narrow areas (color-vision experiments in goldfish, pigeons, and humans; development of the visual system in fish; and experiments on the perception of simple objects), and I found myself reading in areas of vision research that I hadn't even been aware of.

The result of Sandra's work is a book that, as you will see, contains a wealth of information about animal vision—from the perspectives of physics, photochemistry, physiology, anatomy, and psychophysics—but that still fulfills the goal of being entertaining and provocative.

Almost every area of vision research is touched upon in this book, and thus it serves as an introduction to many of the exciting things that are going on in this field of science. Examples include: (1) the understanding of mechanisms of color vision and discrimination, down to the level of individual photopigment molecules and activity in single nerve cells in various parts of the visual system; (2) the processes involved in the development of the visual system, from both the embryological and evolutionary points of view; (3) the study of visual perception as an *active* process, in which the eye and brain most certainly are *not* similar to a passive camera; and (4) the comparative study of unique solutions to visual problems by different species and how we might apply non-human visual abilities in designing modern instruments, such as detection of the plane of polarization of light or the use of mirror optics rather than lenses.

Dean Yeager, Ph.D.
Director
Institute for Vision Research
College of Optometry
State University of New York

Acknowledgments

I owe a special debt to Dean Yager who, without being totally aware of it in the beginning, became my guide throughout this adventure. He gave generously of his time and knowledge throughout the writing of this book. I am exceedingly grateful.

My thanks to Stewart Craig of Bruce Coleman, Inc., a talented photographer in his own right, without whom this book could not have been completed; the staff at Bruce Coleman, Inc.; Gerard Helferich, my editor, who was unfailingly helpful and patient; Margaret Lewis, head librarian, and the rest of the staff at the library of the State University of New York College of Optometry; Mark Meloy, a talented retoucher; my agents, Ivy Fisher Stone, for her persistence and gentle good humor, and Fifi Oscard, ever supportive; and not least, my daughter Meeghan, who likes animals just as much as I do.

Introduction

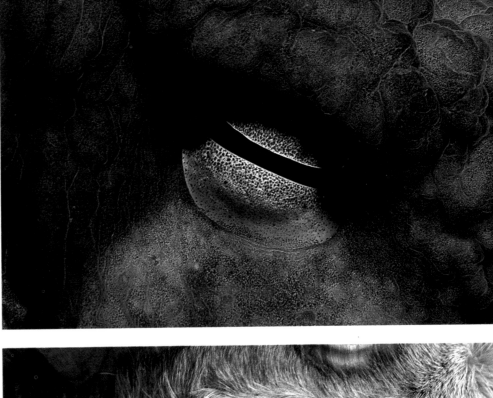

For the vast majority of animals, vision is the most important link to the world. Primitive creatures may be more dependent on their sense of smell, touch or taste, but as we mount the scale of evolution, animals, both predators and prey, rely more and more on their eyes. The eye is the only direct opening of the central nervous system to the world.

From the extraordinary diversity of animal life, it would appear that nature has experimented with all sorts of forms to give her creations a chance to survive in the varied conditions of climate and terrain that are found on this planet. This creativity also extends to the design of the organs of vision. There are eyes on turrets, eyes on tentacles, compound eyes, eyes that see with remarkable clarity in the dark of night or the depths of seas or caves, eyes that can see tapestries of colors that are inaccessible to the human eye. Flowers become vividly marked landing pads for many winged insects, and beetles that appear dull to us are brightly ornamented to their species mates. Pit vipers and boa constrictors have infrared sensing organs that enable them to form heat-sensitive images of enemies and prey. There are a few primitive lizards and fish that have the vestiges of a third eye, known as a pineal eye, on top of their heads. Anyone who has spent a summer's evening in the country is aware that

The pupils of the octopus and squid are rectangular, a shape they share with creatures as dissimilar as bighorn sheep.

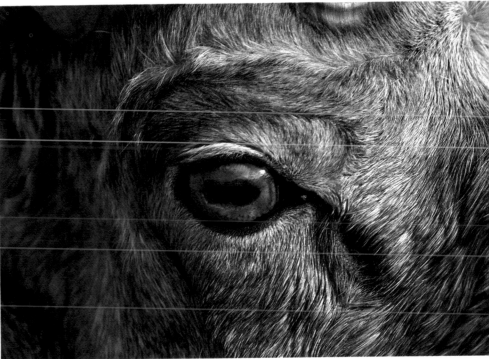

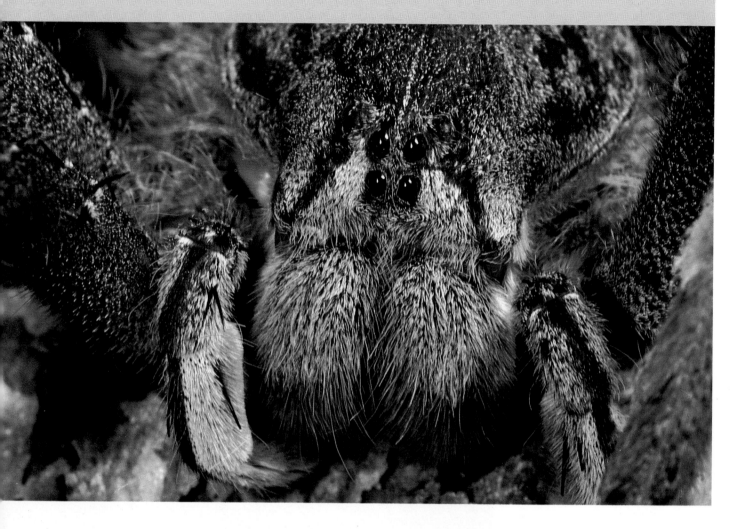

▲

Eyes of the banana spider. All spiders and scorpions have clusters of eyes, generally at least six, but those with the best vision have eight.

there are creatures who can create their *own* light—fireflies. Bioluminescence is also found in other creatures, particularly among marine life; in fact, it becomes crucial to vision as we descend into the depths of the oceans, where no sunlight can penetrate.

Despite this diversity, there is an underlying similarity in the nature of visual perception. All eyes have one thing in common: They are perceivers of light and, in more highly evolved creatures, patterns of light. What we see are not people or plants or other objects themselves but only the light that they reflect or, in the case of bioluminescent creatures, emit.

We all know that plants turn toward the sun, but as any sun-worshiper might guess, all *animal* protoplasm is light-sensitive as well. The first life forms that swam in ancient seas developed patches of light-sensitive cells, allowing them to tell light from dark and even the direction from which the light came. As life evolved, these patches became eyes that could detect first motion, then form, and finally could see the world in brilliant color. Nature is never arbitrary; her gifts have a reason: A creature that can see in color has a better chance of survival.

How a creature sees is determined by three basic factors. The first is whether it is diurnal (that is, awake and active during the day) or nocturnal (awake and active at night) or arrhythmic (capable of activity during the day or night). Second is the creature's environment. Does it live on land or in the sea, or is it airborne? And third is whether it is a creature of prey or a predator.

This third factor has a great deal to do with the position of the eyes in the creature's head. Most predators have their eyes placed squarely in front. (The exception to this rule is predatory fish and deep-sea mammals. How nature compensates them will be discussed in later chapters.) Thus the field of vision of each eye overlaps that of the other, giving the predator great depth perception, the better to pursue its prey. Conversely, creatures of prey have their eyes positioned on the sides of their heads; they have a wide field of view but little binocular vision. Obviously, they have more interest in what might be sneaking up from behind.

A look in the mirror will confirm our worst suspicions about ourselves. We are predators; our eyes are positioned squarely in front of our heads. While primarily diurnal, we can function at night but with limited vision. Our night vision is far inferior to that of the owl. And the eye of the hawk is more accurate than our own during the day. But the eye of the bird has developed at the expense of its brain. (Think of the expression "bird-brained.") This brings us to a most important subject, the crucial role of the brain in interpreting visual signals. Vision is obviously much more than just seeing, even in less-complex forms of life. R. L. Gregory in his book *The Intelligent Eye* even suggests that abstract thinking actually evolved as a result of the eye's effort to make sense of the images it saw.

The smallest creature capable of forming a visual image is the tiny marine copepod the copilia, no larger than the head of a pin. Scientists believe that the copilia is the link between the primitive eyespot and the more complex, image-forming eye. Since the copilia's body is transparent, one can actually see its interior lens, on which two exterior lenses focus light. The interior lens scans back and forth like a television camera, sending signals along a single optic fiber to the brain. As a result, it can take from a fifth of a second to two seconds for a scan to be completed, and only then can the brain construct a complete image. By contrast, think of the rapidity with which we can change focus from the palm of our hand to a distant star.

To the human eye, vision seems instantaneous. The world is simply *there*. Because the human visual mechanism operates at incredible speed, three-hundredths to six-hundredths of a second to form a coherent image during the day and a tenth of a second to form an image at night, we are usually unaware of the visual processing that is taking place.

Successive images flash before our eyes at a rate of 50 to 60 per second during the day and 10 per second at night. That is why a film that moves before our eyes at 24 frames per second appears to be continuous. By contrast, a bee's images move more rapidly, at 300 per second. Thus a motion picture would appear to its eyes as nothing more than a series of still pictures.

Many vision scientists regard the eye as a mini-brain. Of all the organs of sense, only the vertebrate eye is a direct outgrowth of the brain itself.

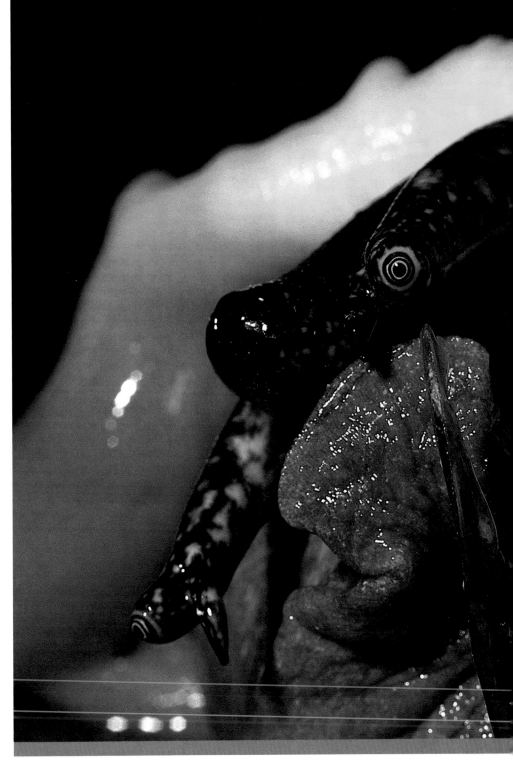

▲

Perched on the ends of tentacles, the eyes of the conch peer out from under the protection of a giant shell.

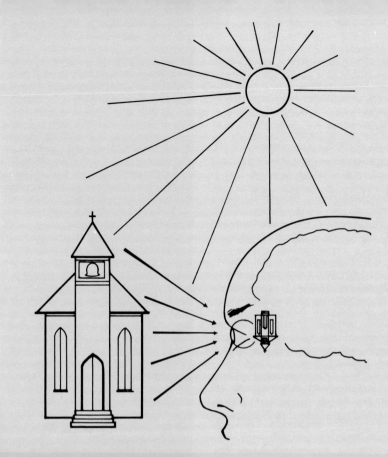

▶ *The retina registers a two-dimensional, upside-down image. It is the brain that transforms these sensations into the sensuous, three-dimensional world with which we are familiar—right-side up, of course.*

▼ *The compound eyes of insects frequently reflect iridescent colors. The star-like pattern in the eye of the goldeneye lacewing is one of the more beautiful examples.*

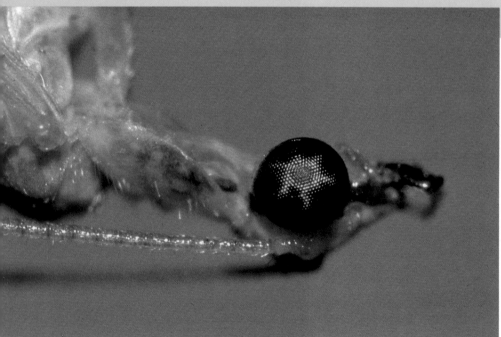

The nerve cells of the eye even resemble those of the brain. In more primitive creatures, much of the information processing is done by the eye itself. However, more advanced creatures actually "see" with their brains, since the trigger cells that respond to specific shapes and colors are found in the visual cortex itself.

But even the human eye edits the visual information that comes to it: Each eye has approximately 130 million photoreceptors, but there are only one million ganglion cells leading to the optic track that forwards the visual signals to the brain. Much of what the eye sees never reaches the brain.

How, in the simplest terms, do we see? The lens of the eye (and in land-dwelling vertebrates, the cornea) bends light waves to focus an image on a screen at the back of the eye (the retina). As you can see from the illustration, the image formed by the vertebrate eye is upside down. From two such upside-down, two-dimensional pictures, the brain forms our image of the world right-side-up and in three dimensions. To me, this is nothing short of miraculous. One has only to think of how perspective works in a painting to get some idea of the work the mind must do to give depth and dimension to what we see. The eye also uses visual clues such as distance and texture to make sense of the images it receives. To realize how important contrast is to the vision of all creatures, consider the stars; they do not actually go out during the day, of course, but all eyes need the dark background of the nighttime sky to perceive them.

The best eyes are able to resolve minute changes in brightness, separating patches of light and dark.

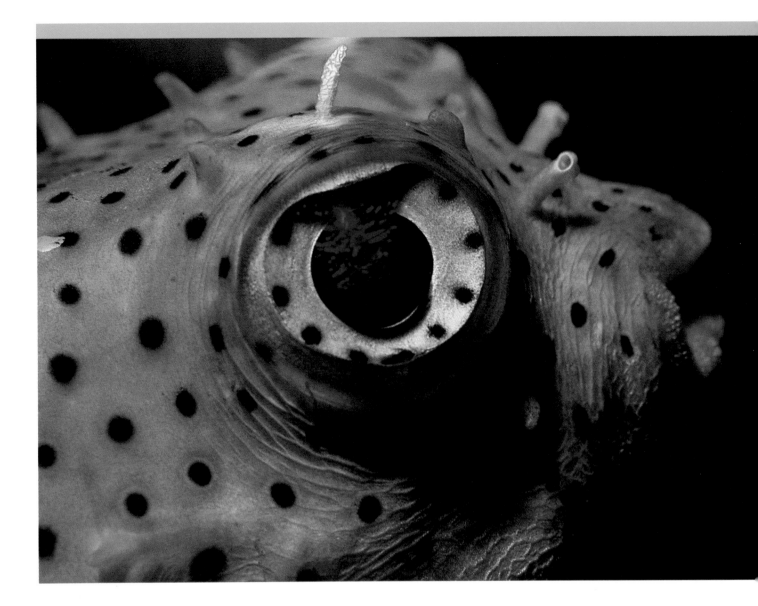

The smaller the difference between light and dark, the more precise the visual image.

Some scientists describe the eye as an imperfect instrument for which the brain must constantly compensate. Many years ago, in experiments conducted by Dr. Anton Hajos of the University of Innsbruck, students wore distorting prismatic lenses that curved straight lines, distorted angles and fringed the outlines of objects with color. After six days of wearing the lenses, the world once again appeared normal to the subjects: The brain had compensated for the distorting lenses. When the students removed the glasses, they again experienced distortions. Again, it took six days for their visual world to return to normal. Similar experiments were performed years later on both chickens and monkeys. Normally, chickens have an innate ability to find seed grains by their shapes; but after the experiment, the hens were completely confused and would have starved to death if left on their own. However, the monkeys were able to adapt: The primate brain seems to be able to assimilate learned behavior even when it contradicts the animal's instincts.

The first eyes could detect only light and dark. The next step in evolution was an eye that could also detect movement. In fact, movement is of major importance to all eyes. The human eye cannot focus on any image for longer than two to three seconds without the image fading. The image must move on the retina or it

The eye of the balloon fish. Patterns of coloration found in the skin of many creatures do not stop at the eye but continue into the corneal covering. This is particularly true of fish, amphibians and reptiles.

will disappear. The human eye jumps every three-tenths to five-tenths of a second in an involuntary tremor that nature seems to have designed to keep our eyes in motion. Although birds cannot move their eyes, they are constantly moving their heads. And while the insect eye is also not mobile, the creature's body is constantly quivering due to heart and respiratory movements. Moreover, if an object moves, the insect is able to see it even more clearly.

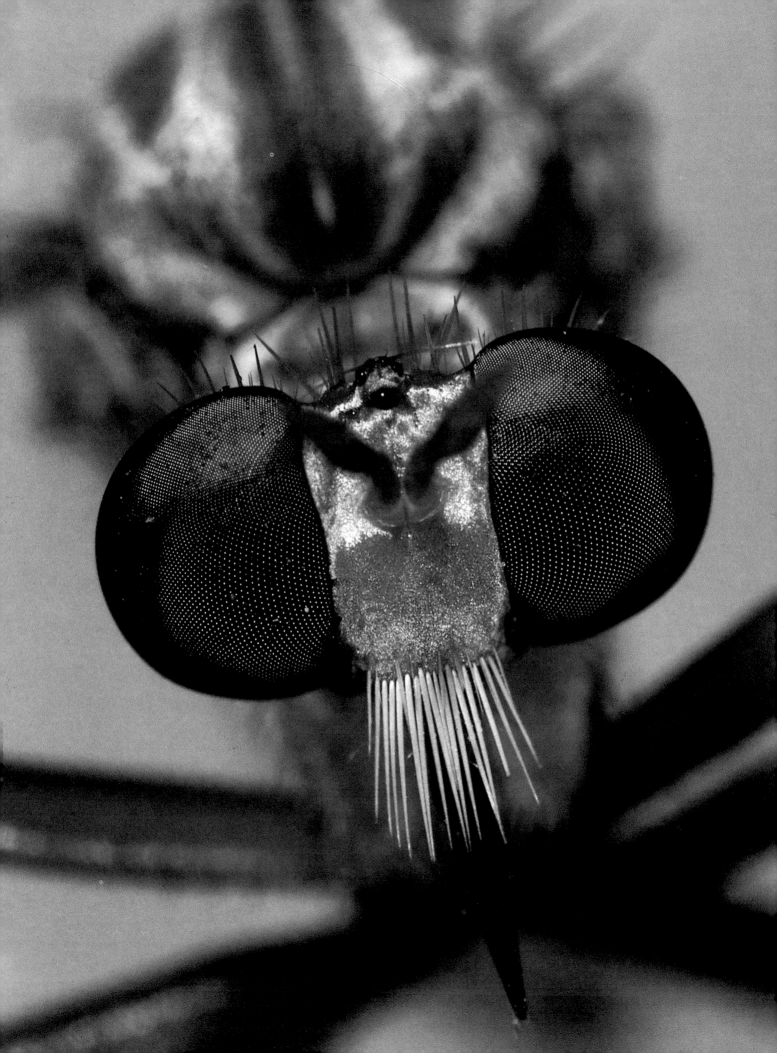

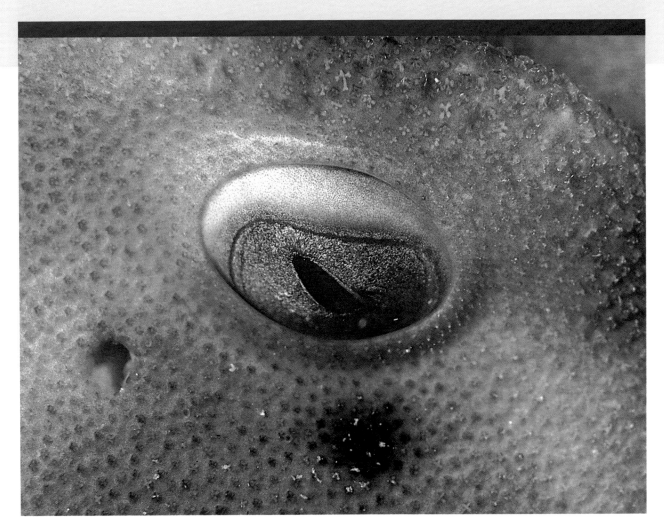

There are limits to vision because eyes can absorb only certain kinds of light. The range of vision in most creatures closely resembles the spectral transmission of light in water, the environment in which life began. The early oceans of the earth acted as a giant filter excluding ultraviolet and infrared radiation. Today, ultraviolet perception is generally found only in flying insects. Perhaps on another world, where evolution began in the atmosphere, there exist creatures with X-ray eyes or infrared vision who are capable of visual perceptions beyond our wildest imagination.

Robber fly. The eyes of most flies are hemispherical in shape, but unlike our own, they are completely free of spherical distortion, which means that the image they see is perfectly clear in all directions.

How is it possible for us to know what animals see, particularly since so much of vision depends on how the brain interprets visual information? Some may argue that we cannot know and that our speculation only exhibits the worst signs of anthropomorphism. However, scientists have spent a great deal of time studying vision and perception in the animal kingdom. There are many practical reasons for these studies. Nature has frequently solved engineering problems that still confound our limited brains. The human eye is nothing more than jelly and sinew, yet its ability to detect contrast far exceeds that of the most sophisticated camera. Similarly, the electric eye owes much of its design to the eye of the frog: What the frog's eye does best is perceive movement. The infrared sensors of snakes can detect changes in temperature in only 35 milliseconds, yet it takes modern instruments almost a full

The eye of the horn shark also has an unusually shaped pupil. Like all fish, it has no lids; these creatures sleep with their eyes open.

minute. Modern mirror telescopes have incorporated some of the design aspects of the eye of the horseshoe crab, whose eye is able to detect varying degrees of contrast, which is of major importance in the study of the night sky.

From these studies has emerged the science of psychophysics, which attempts to bridge the gap between the physics of light and the behavior of living organisms. The advent of the electron microscope in the 1950s enabled scientists to examine individual photoreceptor cells. Structures separated by one-billionth of a meter, a nanometer, can be seen clearly be-

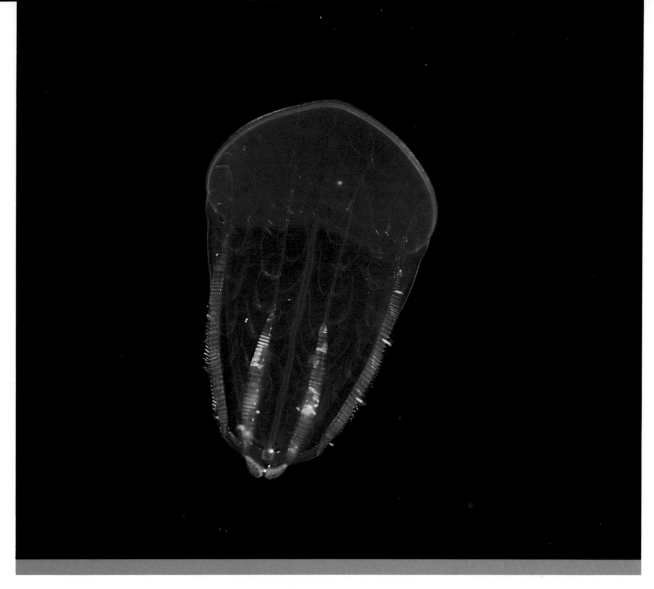

▲

Bioluminescent jellyfish. Many creatures that live beneath the sea can create their own light, as can fireflies and certain bacteria found in fungus. But bioluminescence never occurs in freshwater creatures because it requires the presence of salt.

cause of the extremely short wavelength of the electron. With this technology we can now study the makeup of any creature's eyes in great detail. Sensors can be placed in individual photoreceptor cells that tell us when they "fire." We know which cells are sensitive to color, and even to what colors, and which cells are sensitive only to light intensity. From a study of nerve-cell function, we know which

cells can detect movement, contrast or edging. And from the number of photoreceptors and lenses, we can determine whether the eye can form images or can see only light and shadow.

All this does not mean that there is nothing left to be learned or that there is complete agreement among scientists about the visual capacities of every creature. Despite the explosion of our knowledge of vision, much work remains to be done. But the achievements, particularly in the last twenty-five years, are enormous. Yes, we know that your cat can see colors, though they differ somewhat from the colors you and I see. We know that birds can see the stars; in fact some navigate by the positions of the constellations; and bees can see into the ultraviolet range not discernible to the human eye. All this we know, but can

we actually tell what an animal *sees?* Can we move behind the lenses of other creatures and perceive the world through their eyes? I acknowledge that what we are about to attempt is an educated guess, an adventure of the imaginative mind. But I believe that a leap of the imagination is the beginning of understanding.

Jacob Von Uexkull, a German naturalist, once wondered what it would be like to cross a field of flowers in a bubble. He also wondered what the world looked like to a dog. It is a delight to discover that others have shared my curiosity. And so, in our exploration of how other creatures see, in some cases we will attempt to recreate the vision of some of the other animals with whom we share this planet. Using the photographer's art, we will enter the visual worlds of other creatures.

1

Forming an Image

It is intriguing how the image seen by one creature differs from that seen by another. Primitive creatures respond instinctively to simple shapes; for example, caterpillars climb lines on walls as well as on trees, and small chicks will peck at anything resembling a circle. However, the rich diversity of the human's visual world should not blind us to the value of simpler perceptions that can tell a creature which end is up.

Some modern painters have done us a favor by exploring the simpler strokes that make a more complex pattern. Like the electron microscope, they take us deeper. In the case of vision science, we must enter the realm of the infinitely small if we are truly to understand how all visual images are formed. This is one of the great gifts of modern science, to open for us a level of perception that is ordinarily unavailable to the conscious mind, enabling us to learn from these complex microscopic mosaics how our apparently seamless visual images are constructed.

Nature has evolved three different ways of forming an image. The first is a camera-like eye that brings an image into focus on a continuous receptor surface or screen—the retina. The human eye works on this principle, as do all other eyes in the vertebrate world.

The compound eye is nature's second solution and is found in invertebrates as diverse as the insect, the crustacean and the mollusk. This is a fixed-focus eye with individual refractive units called ommatidia, each responsible for a portion of the visual field. The dragonfly eye has as many

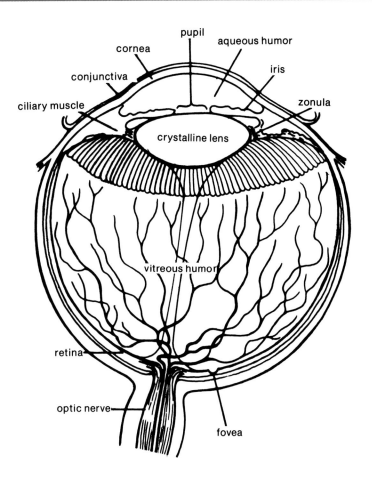

as 28,000 individual ommatidia, giving this insect an almost spherical field of vision. In the case of the compound eye, lens and cornea are one and light is focused by the many small lenses on individual photoreceptors.

The third type of eye scans like a television camera, building a picture from successive impressions. This is the least common form of vision, and one example of it is the already-mentioned copilia.

The eye has been studied for all of recorded history—and perhaps be-

The camera-lens eye. This is a representation of a human eye, which differs little in basic structure from the eyes of all other vertebrates. It has only a single lens.

fore. In some ancient cultures, cataracts were removed from lenses with crude surgical instruments. (If the surgeon blinded a slave, he lost his hand; if he blinded a rich man, he could lose his life. These surgeons must have been men of courage, not

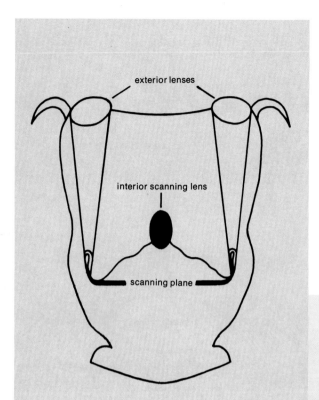

exterior lenses

interior scanning lens

scanning plane

sun   source of light

rays of light entering a single facet of an insect's compound eye

crystalline cone (lens)

pigment

rhabdom

day-active insect

to mention steady hands.) But the importance of the retina to sight is a comparatively late discovery, and it is interesting to note that it was Kepler, the great astronomer—the man who discovered that the planets move around the sun in an elliptical orbit—who first understood the function of the retina as the inner visual screen on which all images are formed.

While eyes may vary in their ability to perceive form, color and movement, all eyes have one thing in common; they are perceivers of light. In fact, it is not *objects* we see, but the light they reflect. While plants do not have eyes, there is a fungus, pilobolus, which, according to Loren Eisley, contains a genuine light-sensitive eye with pigments that control the growth of the fungus' spore cannon and aim it at the area of greatest light. Eisley compares this cannon to a rocket, but what is of greater interest to us is the pigmented depression that follows the movement of the sun. An eye in a plant?

To understand how a visual image is created, we must first begin with the nature of light. Light is one form of energy emitted by the stars of our universe. Newton thought it was composed of particles; later scientists argued that it consisted of waves. After a battle in this century that shook the very foundation of physics, scientists have come to accept that light manifests itself as both a particle and a wave, even though these characteristics are apparently contradictory.

Vision is both an optical and a

chemical process. It will be easier to understand the optical nature of vision by thinking of light as waves and the chemistry of vision by thinking of light as particles.

Light as a Wave

Light forms only a very small portion of the electromagnetic spectrum, whose waves of energy flow throughout the universe, from giant radio waves that may be miles long to the infinitesimally small cosmic rays at the other end of the spectrum. Waves differ from each other in size and frequency of vibration. Larger waves vibrate very slowly, while smaller waves vibrate with extraordinary rapidity. Only wavelength differentiates visible light from other types of electromagnetic energy, such as X-rays, ultraviolet, infrared, and so on.

Visible light ranges from wavelengths of approximately 345 nanometers (billionths of a meter) to approximately 725nm, though no known living creature has vision that encompasses the full range (although tests have shown that certain proteins are sensitive to a wider range of wavelengths, approximately 280nm to 1,000nm). Despite the fact that visible light forms such a small portion of the electromagnetic spectrum, 83 percent of all energy waves that reach the earth fall into this category. Obviously, nature makes use of what is offered. Below 345nm, animal tissue becomes damaged by ultraviolet light, and above 725nm the waves lack the energy to stimulate the photoreceptors of any known eye.

The Optics of Vision

Light travels in a straight line unless it encounters a more dense medium, in which case it is slowed and made to change direction. To the early scientists who studied the nature of light, it appeared to bend; the scientific term is *refraction*. In the sixteenth century it was found that a convex piece of glass could make light rays converge on a point; men soon began to make telescopes and eyeglasses. In effect, they were simply imitating nature's own innovation.

The lens of any eye is a convex prism that bends light and focuses it on the retina. However, in the case of vertebrate land creatures, the cornea is primarily responsible for this function while the lens adjusts the focus for near and far vision. As you can see from the illustration, the image that reaches any retina is upside down; it is the brain, not the eye, that presents the world to us right-side-up.

Waves of light enter the eye from all directions, but not all of them reach the retina. Some are reflected out of the eye. Others are scattered. When a wave of light encounters moisture, it not only changes direction but is also diffused, or dispersed. During the day the sky appears blue because short (blue) wavelengths of light are scattered by our atmosphere. In the morning and evening, the angle at which sunlight strikes the earth changes dramatically and long (red) wavelengths of light are scattered, accounting for our glorious sunrises and sunsets. On a cloudy day, the particles of moisture in the atmosphere tend to be larger, blocking all wavelengths and making the sky appear whiter. The principle of scattering is the same within the eye itself, and the liquid parts of the eye scatter light in the same way. Perhaps no more than 10 percent of all light that reaches a primate eye makes its way to the retina to form an image.

Two other factors that have to do with the optical nature of light will be only mentioned here and discussed in detail later; they are interference and diffraction. Waves of light, like waves of water, tend under certain conditions either to cancel each other out or to reinforce each other. (Interference, by the way, is responsible for one of the great glories of nature, iridescence. The wave nature

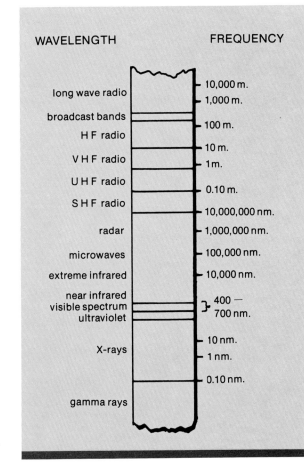

Visible light forms only a very small portion of the electromagnetic spectrum. Wavelengths of visible light differ only in size and frequency of wavelength, from the tiny gamma rays to the giant radio waves.

of light reinforces iridescent colors, giving them a special luster and glow, particularly in the coloration of birds and insects.) Diffraction occurs when a wave must pass through an opening that is smaller than the width of the wavelength. The wave breaks up into smaller rays of light and dark bands or colors. Waves of light that pass through a lens to the retina do not actually converge at a point but form a series of concentric circles of lighter and darker bands. Only larger eyes are able to resolve these bands into one point. This factor is of major importance in the acuity of a visual image; it is also why most insects, with their tiny eyes, can't see stars.

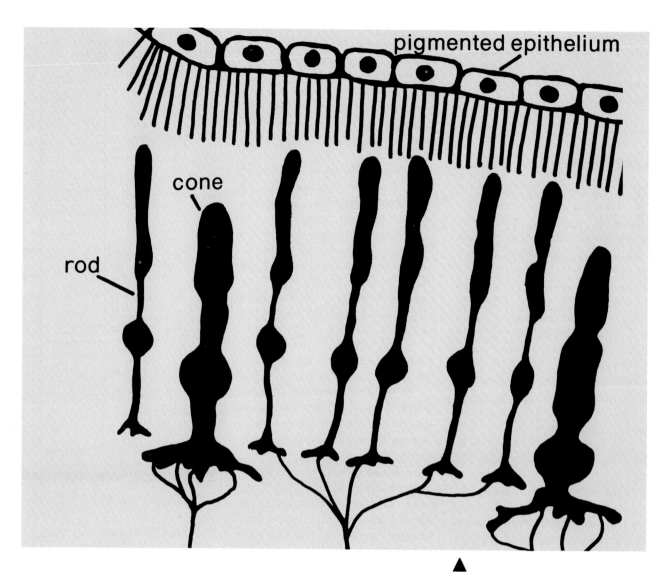

pigmented epithelium

cone

rod

Light as a Particle

It was Einstein's discoveries that caused the great commotion in twentieth-century physics, and he was responsible for calling particles of light *photons*, the basic units of light energy. According to atomic theory, photons originate when electrons are excited by heat and jump from one orbit of an atom to another. If the electron jumps to a nearby orbit, the energy release is comparatively small and the photon vibrates slowly, indicating it has little energy. But if the electron jumps to a far orbit, the emitted photon will vibrate at a high frequency. Thus the eye is constantly being bombarded by photons of varying energy levels.

The speed of light seems to be one of very few constants one can count on in this everchanging world of ours. Its speed, as calculated by modern science, is always 299,792.58 kilometers per second (or about 186,000 miles per second) in a vacuum. Although this fact has become important to scientific calculations only in our century, we have known its approximate speed for several hundred years. Claus Roemer (1644–1710) a Danish astronomer, noted that the eclipses of the four moons of Jupiter are irregular, depending on the distance of Jupiter from the earth. Since Roemer knew that Jupiter is twice the distance of the sun from the earth, he calculated the speed of light at 290,000km per second, which is only about 9,000km off from the measurements made by modern science.

I am sometimes awestruck by

Rods and cones are the photoreceptors of the vertebrate eye. Rods function in dim light and tend to be slender in shape, while cones function in bright light and are generally shorter and thicker. Together they make up the eye's visual screen, called the retina.

the thought that the starlight that guides my path on an evening's walk is millions, even billions, of years old. Yet the photons that strike my eyes arrive undiminished in energy. They are as fresh as the day they were born. If the photon is fortunate enough not to encounter an asteroid, another planet, space debris or particles in our own earth's atmosphere, it will make its way to the surface of the earth, where it can be absorbed by plants or be reflected by inorganic materials, or possibly even make its way into an eye.

The Eye, Perceiver of Light

This is still not the end of the photon's journey, for now it must make its way through the eye. The structures of the compound eye, the vertebrate eye, and the simple invertebrate eye vary to such a degree that they are discussed in separate chapters. But each of these eyes has an outer covering called the cornea, which not only protects the eye but also slows down the light, since the cornea is more dense than air. As the photon is slowed it changes direction. Then it passes through a liquid section, after which it encounters the lens, which is another very dense medium. Again it is slowed and changes direction. If the light is bent in the right direction, the photon will continue on to the retina, where large numbers of light-sensitive cells are waiting to absorb it. However, it may also be reflected right back out of the eye or scattered and made useless for vision by other particles within the eye. Nocturnal creatures have a mirrorlike layer of reflecting cells called a tapetum, which gives the photoreceptors a second chance to receive such scattered photons, thus increasing the nocturnal eye's light-gathering capacities.

The photoreceptors of the invertebrate eye are called rhabdoms. Those of the vertebrate eye are separated into rods and cones. Rods function in dim light and are also important to peripheral vision, while cones react to brighter light and are responsible for discriminating colors.

The Photochemistry of Vision

Both the rods and cones of vertebrate photoreceptors and the rhabdoms of invertebrates contain visual pigment, in the molecules of which the absorption of photons takes place. There is more than one type of visual pigment.

Visual pigment molecules, called chromoproteins, are combinations of large protein molecules called opsin and a form of carotenoid pigment called retinene. The main characteristic of carotenoids is that they bend. In fact, they bend themselves around the opsin molecule, linking together in what is known in chemistry as the *cis* position. But when the large chromoprotein molecule absorbs a photon, it causes the carotenoid to straighten out, and the large molecule falls away from the opsin. They are then in the *trans* position.

There are a number of different types of visual pigment. When fused, the carotenoid and the opsin assume different colors depending on the type

▼

Before absorbing a photon of light, the chromophore and opsin form one giant molecule in the 11-cis configuration. But once the photon is absorbed, the visual-pigment molecule disintegrates until it can again be reconstituted by the absorption of a form of Vitamin A_1 or A_2.

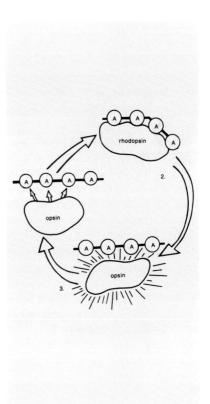

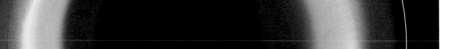

Prismatic diffraction. One reason insects cannot see distant stars is that vibrating photons kick off the edges of the lenslets and do not land in a single point on the photoreceptors but in a series of concentric circles, thus blurring the image.

of retinene present. In fact, this coloration is sometimes visible in the eyes of animals. For example, rhodopsin, the most common form of visual pigment, is rose-colored; porphyropsin, found in freshwater fish, is deep purple; and deepsea fish have a golden visual pigment that is most sensitive to blue wavelengths. When the molecule separates, it is said to have "bleached," and the retinene by itself appears yellowish.

This basic process is common to the vision of all living creatures. What chlorophyll is to photosynthesis, carotenoids are to photoreception. However, animals cannot make carotenoids themselves, but must ingest it from plants. That's why your mother told you to eat your carrots.

Ingested carotenoids are transformed by enzymes into a usable form called either retinal or retinol, which is a form of Vitamin A_1 or Vitamin A_2 and which is stored in the liver for future use. People who suffer from night blindness may be deficient in Vitamin A. Predatory nocturnal cats are known to eat the liver of their prey first, and although the ancient Egyptians knew nothing of Vitamin A, they did know that eating liver could cure night blindness.

In the case of vertebrates, the chromoprotein molecule must re-form itself so that it can again absorb photons; it revitalizes itself with some form of Vitamin A_1 or A_2. Once more the carotenoid curves around the protein molecule and they again assume the *cis* position. (Some invertebrates go through an intermediate state in re-forming, which will be discussed in detail in another chapter.)

▶

Pathways to the brain, vertebrate eye. Light is first absorbed by the individual photoreceptors and transformed into electrical energy that is transmitted by two layers of nerve cells in the eye itself, the bipolars and the ganglion cells, before the visual information is sent on to the brain via the optic nerve. Note that the photoreceptors face the brain rather than the incoming light.

Pathways to the Brain

The optical picture formed on the retina is only the beginning of perception. In fact, higher vertebrates can be said to see with their brains. An eye may function perfectly, but if the visual cortex of the brain is destroyed, the creature will not be able to see and will suffer from what is called "blind sight." On the other hand, creatures lower on the evolutionary scale process more information within the eye itself, and therefore even if a portion of the visual part of their brain is removed, these creatures may still retain some sight.

The first group of cells to receive visual information from the photoreceptors is the bipolar cells. In a vertebrate eye that has both rods and cones (there are some creatures with either pure rod or almost-pure cone vision), the number of rods connected to each bipolar cell is far greater than the number of cones connected to each. As a result, the cone photoreceptors are said to have a more direct line of communication. (If you think of an operator listening on a line where many people are trying to speak at the same time, you'll get some idea of what I mean.) Rod information is described as being summed or pooled. But rods require less light stimulation

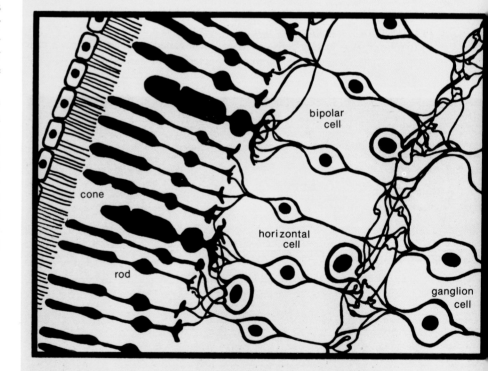

than cones, and dominant rod vision is found in nocturnal or crepuscular creatures. (Crepuscular creatures are those generally active at dawn or dusk.) Creatures with dominant cone vision are diurnal, generally functioning during the day.

At the bipolar level, impulses from the photoreceptors are either inhibited or sent on to a third layer called the ganglion cells. Running parallel to the bipolar and ganglion cells are horizontal and amacrine cells, which may aid in the inhibition of information and the clearing of the visual map.

At each level, there are fewer nerve cells to pass information forward. For example, the human eye contains as many as 130 million photoreceptor cells, but there are only around 1 million ganglion cells. From this we can deduce the extraordinary amount of processing done by the eye itself. No wonder so many scientists refer to the eye as a ''mini-brain.'' Until this point, the basic chain described here is common to most creatures.

From the ganglion cells, visual information is sent on to the brain via the optic fibers. Since the visual areas of the brain vary in complexity, they will be discussed in detail as we consider each group of animals. In lower vertebrates and most invertebrates, much of the visual processing is done by the eyes. These creatures tend to have instinctive responses determined by shape, size and sometimes color. Their visual systems are dominated by trigger cells, that is, cells that respond to specific stimuli. Cells in the eyes of higher vertebrates, in contrast, are nonselective until one reaches the brain, but here the com-

Pathways to the brain, compound eye. In the case of the invertebrate eye, the photoreceptor cells face the direction of the incoming light. Cornea and lens are one, though the light must travel down the path of a lens cylinder, which varies in length among invertebrates.

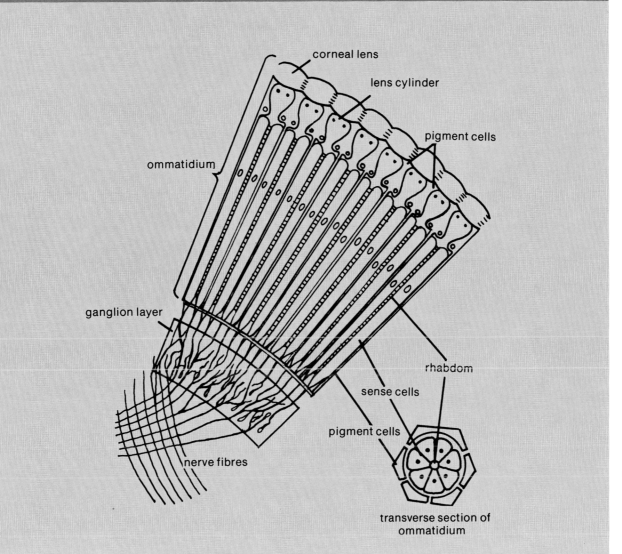

corneal lens

lens cylinder

pigment cells

ommatidium

ganglion layer

rhabdom

sense cells

pigment cells

nerve fibres

transverse section of ommatidium

plexity becomes truly awesome. De Valois in his studies of the macaque monkey has shown that some cells in the visual area of this creature's brain respond only to a shadow on a very small area of the back of its hand.

In visual systems dominated by trigger cells, form vision is less developed, and these creatures are better at determining size or location. Even color vision may be discriminated at a lower level of brain activity, but form vision or the ability to recognize complex patterns is an activity of the higher brain centers.

Less is known about the visual connections in the compound eye. In most cases the compound eye is so small that until recently it has been extremely difficult to examine the neural connections to the brain.

Patterns of Light—the Visual Image

Since a visual image is nothing more than a pattern of light, one of the basic properties of the visual system is its sensitivity to contrast, the ability to detect an edge or a contour, which is determined by a change in lightness and darkness across the visual field.

First, the eye adapts itself to the average level of light available. Everything above this level reads as brighter, everything below as darker. The receptor surface of the retina is frequently described as a mosaic of photoreceptors. It is possible to compare this layer to film emulsion. Fine-grain film makes a precise, highly accurate image or photograph; similarly, a retina with many, tightly packed photoreceptors gives an eye a very distinct picture of the world around it. One of the reasons for the keen vision of the hawk is the density of the cones packed into its retina; there are over 1 million cones per square inch.

Color vision makes an animal more sensitive to changes in contrast, a potentially life-saving capacity. What we call a change in color is actually a change in wavelength: The shortest wavelengths fall in the ultraviolet, and the longest wavelengths are red. In between there is a large number of hues, though we generally speak of the basic colors as violet, blue, green, yellow, orange and red. The trained human eye can discern as many as 150 hues, while a freshwater fish such as the perch may be able to discriminate only about 26, but both have their limitations: Fish cannot see into the blue area of the spectrum, while the normal human eye cannot see into the near ultraviolet. The greatest sensitivity of the human eye occurs at about 555nm, which just happens to be the shade of yellow-green that matches the forest canopy, which should tell us something about our distant past as forest creatures. Bees can see into the ultraviolet range and are most sensitive between 480 and 510nm, yet they cannot see reds, while marine fish that live in the deepest oceans are more sensitive to the blue area of the spectrum—about 490nm.

Limits define. They can also enrich. Creatures with eyes limited in spectral sensitivity or focal length may see greater detail or variety of color within that narrower range. Butterflies, for instance, see details in flowers that are lost to our eyes, and flies, while more limited in spectral sensitivity, can distinguish more hues than we can within their area of greatest sensitivity.

The visual image, the pattern of light that is passed on to the brain and stored in the form of visual memory, enables animals to recognize objects, identify them and learn. Vision scientists tell us that even some of the simplest creatures have "sameness" neurons and "newness" neurons, nerve cells that can separate images that have been seen before from those that are new. How awesome are the complex interactions that make up a single glance.

2

Primitive Eyes

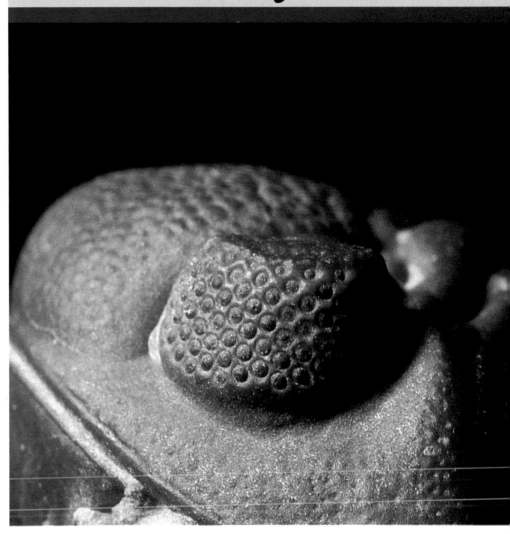

There is greater diversity in the vision of invertebrates than in that of vertebrates. (An invertebrate is an animal without an internal skeleton or backbone.) We vertebrates are apt to sneer at the spineless, but some invertebrates have remarkable vision. The largest classification in the animal kingdom, with over one million species—more than double the number of vertebrates—invertebrates include creatures as diverse as sponges, jellyfish, starfish, mollusks, insects, spiders and crustaceans. Yet all these creatures have common visual elements. Despite the dissimilarity of their appearance, insects and cephalopods (mollusks like octopi and squid) have eyes with a similar photoreceptor design.

Yet within this group we find the pigment depressions that serve as eyes for the earthworm as well as the largest eye of any animal, that of architeuthis, the giant squid. To get an idea of its size, consider that the diameter of the human eye is a mere 3cm, while that of the giant squid is about 370cm; the giant squid have exceptional vision. In the next four chapters, we will explore the vision of invertebrates as diverse as spiders, crustaceans, insects and cephalopods, but first something about primitive eyes.

The oldest eye of which we have any record belongs to the trilobite. From fossilized remains, we know that this ancient marine creature which lived 500 million years ago had a compound, faceted eye that could see to the side but not up. Yet nature allows us a living glimpse of this past: The larva of another ancient creature that has managed to survive to the present day, limulus, the horseshoe

crab (a crustacean so old that its blood is based on copper rather than iron) resembles the long-extinct trilobite.

The larvae and fetuses of animals tell us much about the history of the species. There is a saying in biology that phylogeny follows ontogeny, meaning that we see in the fetus or larva the racial history of that species. The gill slits of the human embryo testify to our past in the sea. The eyes of the seal fetus emerge at the

▲

Eye of trilobite. Fossilized remains of trilobites reveal a compound eye that saw clearly around, but not up.

front of its head, a reminder of its days as a land predator, and move toward the side of the head before birth. Even the larvae of blind cave fish have eyes, though they disappear upon maturity, telling us that their ancestors were sighted.

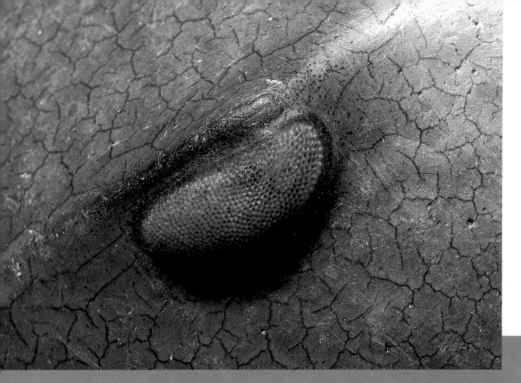

◀

The horseshoe crab is so ancient that its blood is based on copper rather than iron. It has both compound eyes and simple eyes, although it relies primarily on the compound eyes for image formation.

▼

Two bat starfish stare at one another through the eyes in their feet. Below we see a close-up of the light-sensitive photoreceptors in the foot.

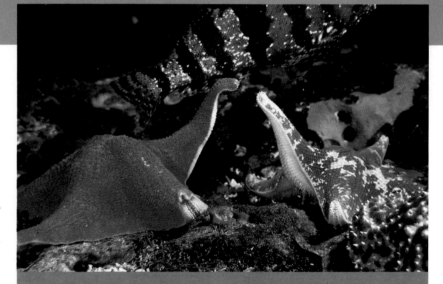

The Photosensitivity of Primitive Creatures

The entire bodies of primitive invertebrates such as jellyfish, coral, sea anemones, worms, starfish and sea urchins are sensitive to light. Their primitive eyes are nothing more than a collection of eyespots or photosensitive cells, and even if these eyes are covered, their bodies remain light-sensitive.

The eyes of the earthworm are pigmented depressions covered by a transparent jelly. In jellyfish, the eyespots are raised patches of cells. In echinoderms (such as starfish and sea urchins), eyespots are found at the end of a foot or tentacle. All these eyes not only distinguish light from dark but also sense the direction from which the light is coming. As evolution proceeded, the patches of photosensitive cells became indented and were covered by a transparent layer of skin that became the lens. Photoreceptor cells became more numerous and formed a retina. Screening pigment formed a protective layer beneath the retina so that light could not escape into the rest of the body.

Primitive Eyes

10

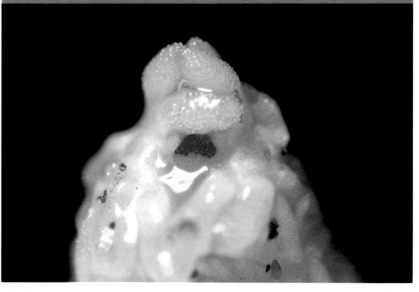

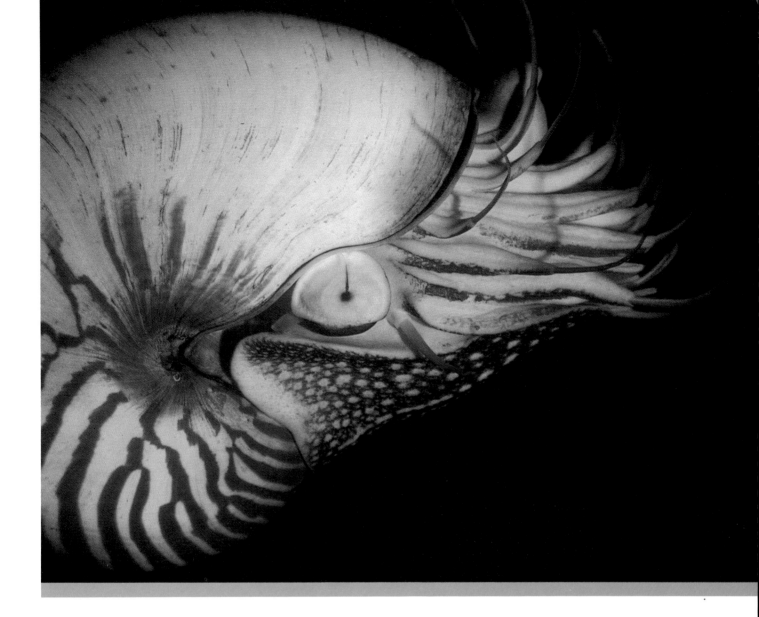

Simple Mollusks

One creature whose photoreceptors are indented but who did not develop a lens is the chambered nautilus. The nautilus is interesting not only for its beauty but because it is a cephalopod, a type of mollusk that includes creatures with such advanced vision that they will be considered separately. The nautilus, however, is a more primitive example. It is also the only cephalopod to possess a shell, which is used for buoyancy as well as protection from predators. The vision of the nautilus is based on the same principle as the pinhole camera. Early cameras did not have lenses and used only a pinhole to focus an image. Like these primitive cameras, the nautilus requires a great deal of light to get an image of any quality.

Two other mollusks with interesting visual mechanisms are the cone shell and the spider shell, both found on tropical reefs all over the world. These animals' eyes are positioned on raised stalks called ommatophores, each of which also has an olfactory and a tactile node. The stalk is held rigid by a series of muscles that also enable it to be withdrawn into the shell when necessary.

These creatures are the most primitive invertebrates able to move their lenses in order to focus more clearly. When the stalk is fully engorged, pressure is placed on the back of the eyes, altering their axis and their focal length and enabling the animals to change focus. Both the cone shell's

The chambered nautilus has no cornea or lens covering, so its vision is best compared to that of a pinhole camera.

and the spider shell's eyes have no iris or pupil. While the creatures can change color to match their background, it is not known if they can *see* color.

Primitive mollusks never have just one simple eye. Some have hundreds of eyes, like the frond worm, or rows of eyes, like the scallop. While these creatures may not see clear images, they are very sensitive to movement. The scallop will remain open to very slow movements and even rapid ones, but if the movement approximates the speed of a creature

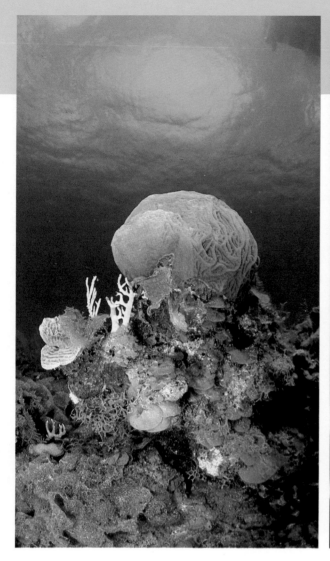

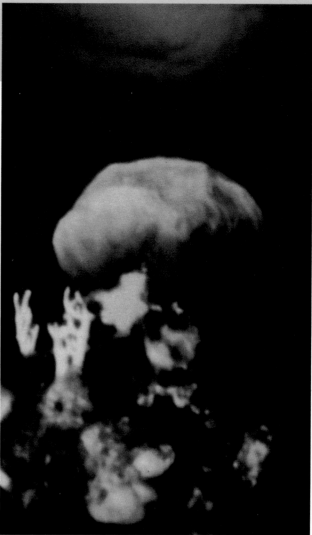

who preys upon it (such as the whelk or the starfish), the scallop shuts immediately.

Eyeshine

This is a widespread phenomenon in the animal world, particularly among nocturnal creatures and fish. Eyeshine is produced by a layer of reflecting cells, called a tapetum, that captures photons that might otherwise escape and reflects them back on the retina, increasing the animal's ability to see clearly in the dark. In the case of the scallop, the reflecting layers of the tapetum are made of a crystalline substance called guanine which gives the eyes a mirrorlike quality.

The tapetum may also enable the scallop to form some sort of image.

Until fairly recently, it was thought that the scallop could only tell light from dark and detect movement, since the scallop's lens does not focus an image on its retina. This is a common problem in the animal world. We all know people who are farsighted (where the image is focused in front of their retinas) or nearsighted (where the image is focused behind their retinas). They need additional lenses, in the form of eyeglasses or contacts, to correct their vision. But the lens of the scallop actually focuses the image outside the creature's eye. Scallops obviously cannot wear rows of glasses, but nature may have provided them with another corrective means.

In 1966, a scientist named M. F. Land concluded that the tapetum of the scallop actually reflects light

▲

Here we see a reef both as we would view it and how it might be seen by a chambered nautilus. Since their lens aperture is so small, there is excellent depth of field, but the visual image is very dim in contrast to our own.

back onto the far side of the retina, which is spherical in shape and parallel to the tapetum. This would mean that the scallop could receive a reflected image on the retina and could discern forms of some sort, though how clearly is questionable. This is the only case I know of where tapetums are thought to serve any function other than capturing more light.

Primitive Photoreceptors

Photoreceptor cells vary from species to species, but all have developed from one of nature's original creations, the cilium. Anyone who has looked at protozoa under a microscope has seen these creatures propel themselves with waving cilia or flagella. Nature has modified cilia into a wide variety of shapes to form chemical, mechanical and light receptors. Some have been folded over and over again to form discs or have been flattened into membranes to form a sac. The scallop has ciliary sacs in its rows of eyes. There are other shapes: lamellae, microbutues, villi, etc. The photoreceptors of most primitive creatures are villi. Structurally, these ciliary shapes vary from species to species, but they all serve a similar purpose. In primitive creatures the villi are disorganized and the shapes quite tortuous. These are the creatures who can simply detect light from dark.

Molecules of visual pigment do not just cluster or hang in space but are suspended from the sides of the photoreceptors. As creatures evolve, the photoreceptors become more organized in layers or rows of cells. In the most advanced invertebrates, the layers of microvilli are found in perpendicular layers or rows, which enables them to detect polarized light. As a result, creatures such as cephalopods or bees are able to ascertain the angle at which their photoreceptors are struck by light and thus the position of the sun no matter what the weather. Both bees and cephalopods are excellent navigators. Keep in mind that the detection of polarized light is not something they have to figure out; they know it in the same way that we know the sky is blue.

Some of the more primitive mollusks that are able to detect polarized light have very poor form vision. In the watery world of most mollusks, where light is polarized by the molecules of water through which they must pass, any improvement in vision can have important survival value. With sharks and whales and the many other predators who feed on them, mollusks deserve all the help they can get.

Scallops are better at detecting movement than at forming an image. If an object moves with the speed of one of their predators, such as the whelk, the scallops shut immediately.

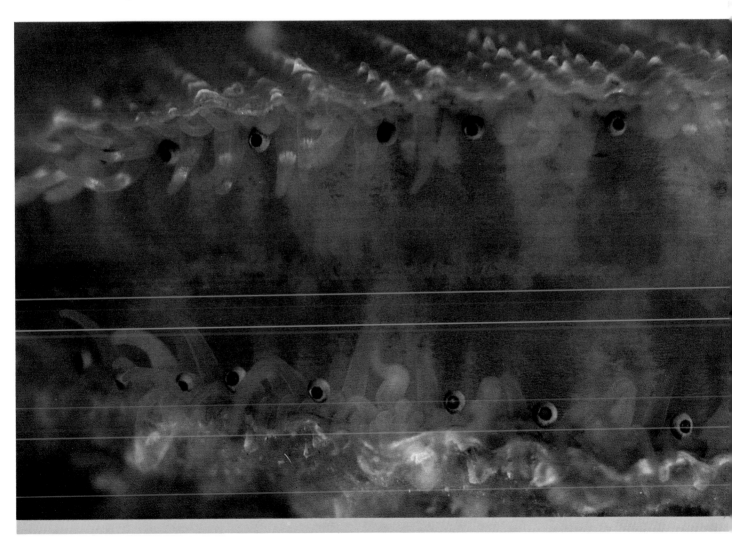

3 *Spiders*

Scorpions date from Devonian times. That's at least 350 million years ago. Spiders appeared around 50 million years later. At that time, there were no birds, no mammals, and no flying insects except for some clumsy ant lions or doodlebugs. Flies came along some 100 million years later, in the Jurassic period. Arachnids, i.e., spiders and scorpions, were already clearly differentiated long before man was even a gleam in Mother Nature's eye. And their visual organs were much the same then as they are today.

Both spiders and scorpions have what are called simple eyes, which is only a way of distinguishing them from the compound eyes of other invertebrates. There is nothing simple about them. In the first place, neither creature ever has just one eye but always has a cluster of eyes, usually six to eight. The visual mechanisms of both are remarkably similar, though scorpions are always nocturnal while some spiders are diurnal (including the jumping spider, which is considered to have the best vision of any arachnid). Also scorpions, unlike spiders, are confined to warmer climes. One characteristic both share is that they become temporarily blind when they shed their hardened exterior skeletons for new ones. This molting is common to all Arthropoda—crustaceans, insects and arachnids.

There is considerable variation in quality of vision among spiders. However, those that do see well have some color vision and also the capacity to see polarized light. The largest simple eye of all spiders belongs to an Australian nocturnal species called the net-casting spider; the strangest belongs to the male midget spider,

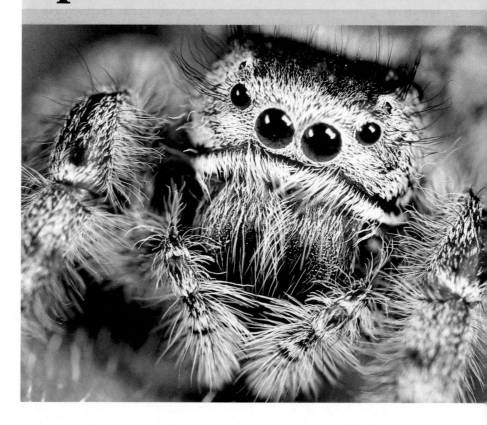

▲

The eight-eyed jumping spider has the best vision of the arachnids. The two pairs of eyes on the sides of the head perform a similar function to our own peripheral vision. The smaller pair of frontal eyes act as distance estimators, while the larger main eyes form the image.

whose eyes are perched on the ends of stalks.

Spiders are divided into weavers and hunters. The weaver can wait for the web to do its work, but the hunting spider must catch its prey, and that undoubtedly is why nature has given it better eyesight.

The Jumping Spider

Jumping spiders have the best vision of all the hunting spiders. They are very small, about 7mm wide, and some of them are quite hairy. But if you can get close enough, you will note the intensity of their stare. They have a total of eight eyes that divide all the functions we associate with one eye: peripheral vision, distance estimation and image formation. The two large front eyes are the most important in forming an image. These are called the main, or anterior median, eyes. On either side of the main eyes are two smaller eyes, the anterior lateral, and then on either side of the head, two additional sets called the posterior median eyes and the posterior lateral eyes. The two sets of eyes on either side of the head are much smaller and service the spider's peripheral vision; they are detectors of motion rather than images.

Like all other spiders, the jumping spider has no lens accommodation. That is, it cannot switch from near to far vision, but, depending on an object's distance, must either move closer to or farther away from it in order to see the object clearly. How then can it capture its prey or avoid being eaten by birds, wasps, praying mantis, lizards and the many other predators that feed on it? After all, the species has managed to sur-

▼
How a horsefly might appear to a jumping spider. The spider's best image formation occurs at about eight to ten centimeters away.

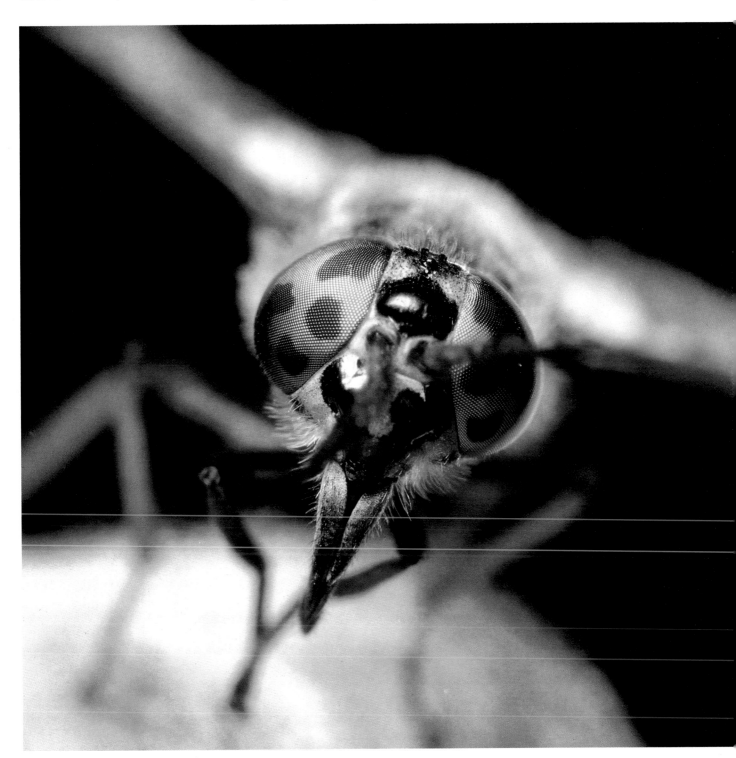

vive a very long time. The answer is that they can see very well within a limited area; and then, of course, jumping spiders can jump.

The maximum distance that any spider can see is 30 to 40 centimeters, or roughly a foot, though the jumping spider's best image formation occurs at 8 to 10 centimeters away. Most spiders will not jump at a prey till it is 3 to 4 centimeters, or a little more than an inch, away. But there is one hunting spider, *Altus saltator,* that can jump 20 times its own length, granted that it is only 3 centimeters long.

The vision of the jumping spider has been described as similar to that of a telephoto lens—excellent within a limited area. Now, even though this spider cannot use its lens to accommodate for near or far vision, nature allows it to compensate for its narrow angle of view by shifting the retina itself up, down, and sideways, greatly increasing the field of vision.

With its secondary eyes posi-tioned on the sides of its head, the jumping spider can see the move-ments of an insect several inches away. It will then turn and focus its four frontal eyes on its prey. The smaller of the frontal eyes have a wider range of vision and judge distance; the main eyes are used to form the im-age. If the image is unclear, the spi-der will move closer for a better look.

Jumping spiders communicate with one another using visual signs. Male wolf spiders use their arms like semaphores, sending signals to pro-

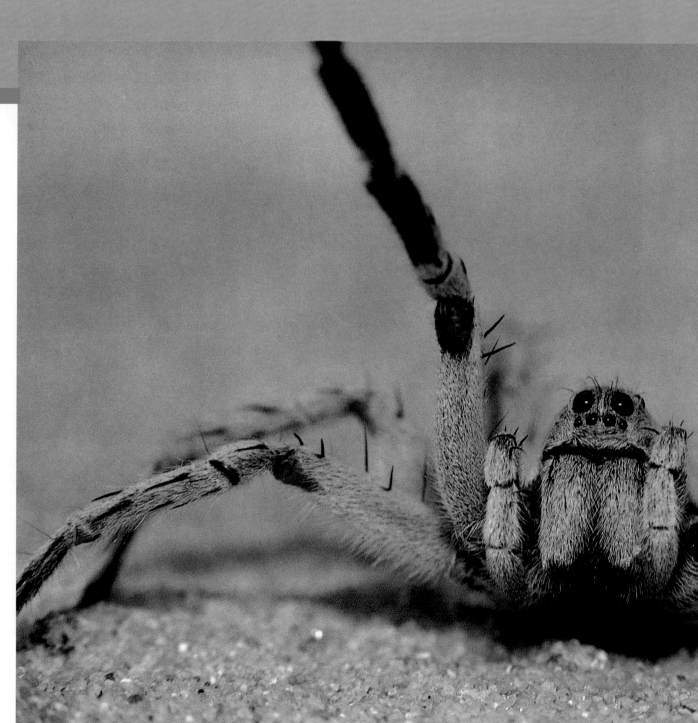

spective mates or threatening other males. In addition to jumping, *Altus saltator* likes to pirouette from side to side during courtship. Moreover, many jumping spiders have ultraviolet markings that can only have significance for other members of the species.

The wolf spider also has excellent vision and is known to send visual signals using its arms as semiphores.

Some Variations in Spiders' Eyes

The spherical lenses of the main eyes ensure images of high quality. These eyes are quite black in appearance, since they lack the tapetal cells that reflect light. The eye is composed of a lens, which is a jellylike body; behind this are the photoreceptor cells and the visual pigment that absorbs light.

The photoreceptor cells are called rhabdoms rather than rods or cones. In all invertebrates, the rhabdoms are structurally the same whether or not they function for color or monochromatic vision. (Rods and cones, in contrast, are morphologically distinct.) We know that an invertebrate can possess color vision when there are at least two types of visual pigment present in the rhabdoms with different peak-wavelength sensitivities.

Generally, the photoreceptors of all invertebrates face outward toward the lens in the direction of the

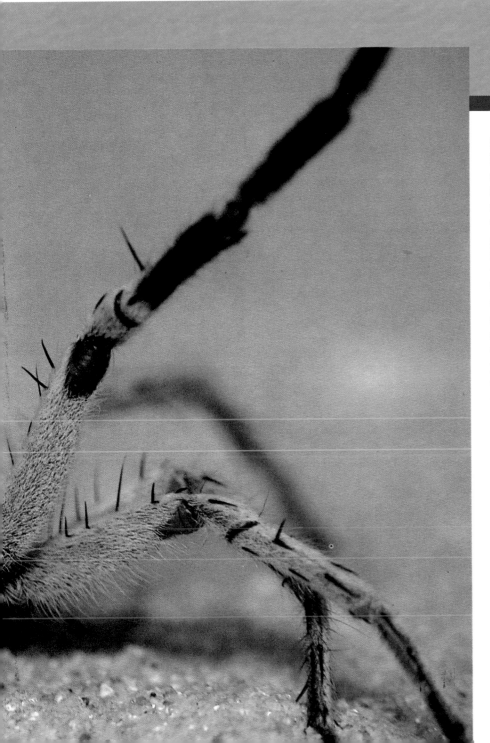

incoming light, while those of vertebrates face away from the lens in the direction of the brain. This difference is important and is based on the animal's evolution. The retina of the vertebrate is thought to be an outgrowth of the brain while that of the invertebrate has evolved from an invaginated bubble in the skin. On the basis of this fact, science has concluded that vertebrates do not descend from invertebrates but have had a separate evolution. The two types of retinas even connect to different parts of the brain. Retinas that face outward in the direction of the incoming light are described as unreversed while those that face the brain are called reversed. The spider is unusual in that it has both reversed and unreversed retinas. (This is a characteristic it shares with another invertebrate, the scallop, which also has both types of retinas, but each in a different row of eyes.)

The main eyes of spiders are typically invertebrate; the retinas face in the direction of the incoming light, but the retinas of the secondary eyes are reversed and face away from the lens. Unlike the main eyes, the secondary eyes also possess a reflecting

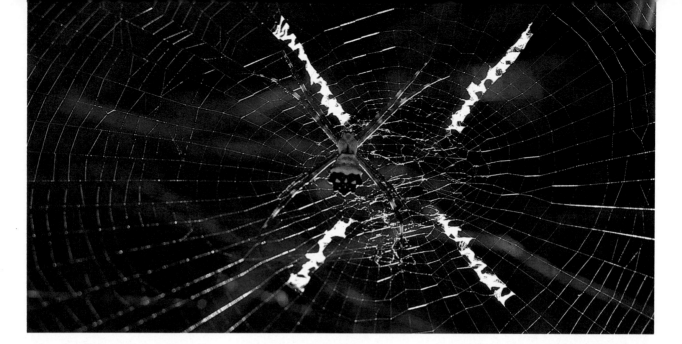

layer, or tapetum, that enables them to absorb more light. Since these eyes are primarily detectors of motion, that extra sensitivity is a distinct asset.

The main eyes of spiders tend to be rather uniform in structure, but the secondary eyes vary widely from species to species. There are three types of secondary eyes. In the most primitive, the tapetum fills the entire cup, leaving holes for other fibers. In another, the tapetum is described as canoe-shaped, and in the third, which is also the most efficient, the tapetum resembles a grate. The structure of this tapetum is more ordered, typical of the dictum that the more evolved a structure, the greater its organization.

The main eyes of spiders are not always found in front, and the position of the eyes is important in classifying spiders. However, the main eyes of jumping spiders are always the anterior median (front middle), while the main eyes of another hunter, the wolf spider, are located on the side—either the posterior lateral eyes or the posterior median eyes—and the four frontal eyes are very small. The main eyes of most spiders are actually very small; the jumping spider along with the crab spider are diurnal exceptions, while the net-casting spider of Australia is a nocturnal exception. Spiders with only six eyes have no main eyes at all. These include the daddy longlegs and all weaving spiders.

Weaving Spiders

For nonhunting spiders, vision is not important, but orb weavers can detect changes in light intensity and will drop from their webs if approached. Moreover, even though the orb weaver's own sight is limited, it weaves large visual signs, called stabilimenta, into its web to warn away birds and other large creatures that might otherwise stumble through and break them. The spider takes a calculated risk of also warning away creatures that it normally preys upon, such as butterflies, in order to preserve its web.

The Net-Casting Spider

This is undoubtedly the most unusual of all nocturnal spiders, most of whose vision is very poor. It is not that its eyes have the ability to form a sharp image; in that respect the vision of the jumping spider is far superior. But its lens has the extraordinary ability to concentrate light on the retina. In their studies of this spider, A. D. Blest and M. F. Land suggest that its lens resembles that of a fish and is one of the few lenses to be totally free of any spherical aberration or color distortion. Composed of concentric materials whose refractive index decreases from the center to the

▲

While the vision of weaving spiders is not as good as that of hunting spiders, they are well aware of the importance of vision to other creatures and weave warning signs called stabilimenta into their webs to avert their destruction by birds or large insects.

The eyes of the female net-casting spider of Australia are the largest of any spider and have a remarkable ability to capture photons—as many as 2,000 times the number absorbed by the eye of the jumping spider or even the human eye.

periphery, the gradient is so exact that all light rays entering the eye can be brought into focus at one point.

The net-casting spider has the largest eyes of any spider and each eye can absorb 2,000 times as many photons as the jumping spider at night; all this without any tapetum. Its eyes have an f-stop of 0.58, and that's what any photographer would call a very fast lens.

Another anomaly is that the net-casting spider is a weaver. However, this spider does not sit and wait for its prey to come along; it weaves its web and then drops it on unsuspecting prey like a net. Only the female of this species can weave the net, and her eyes are far larger than the eyes of the male.

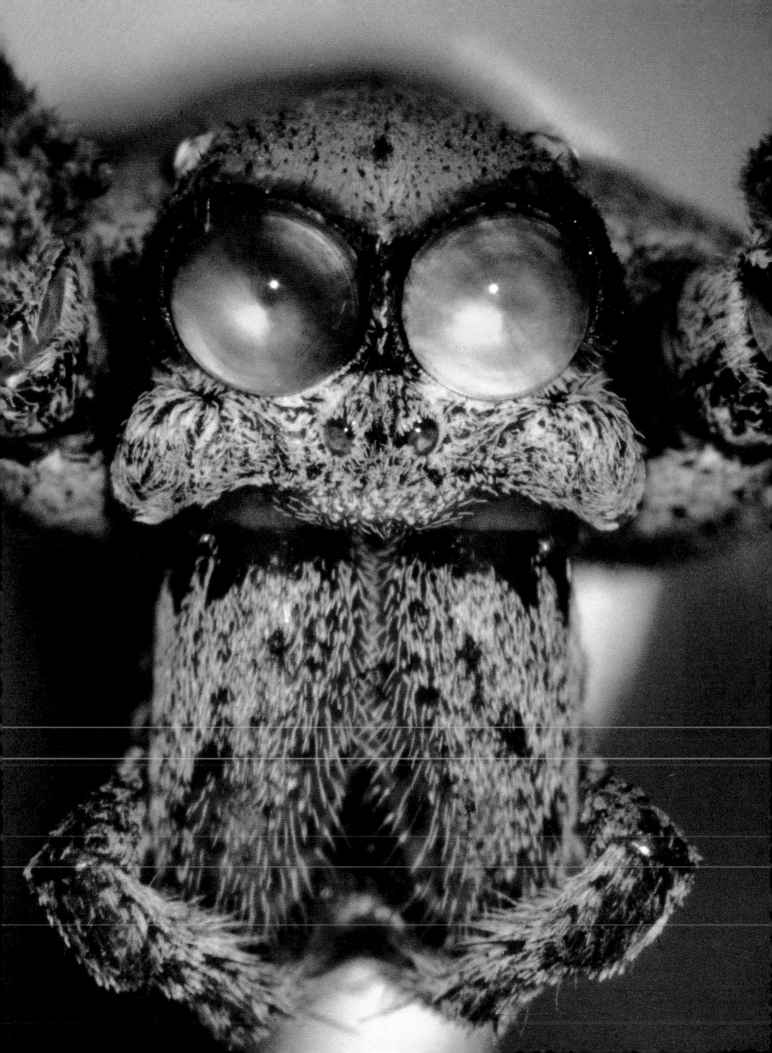

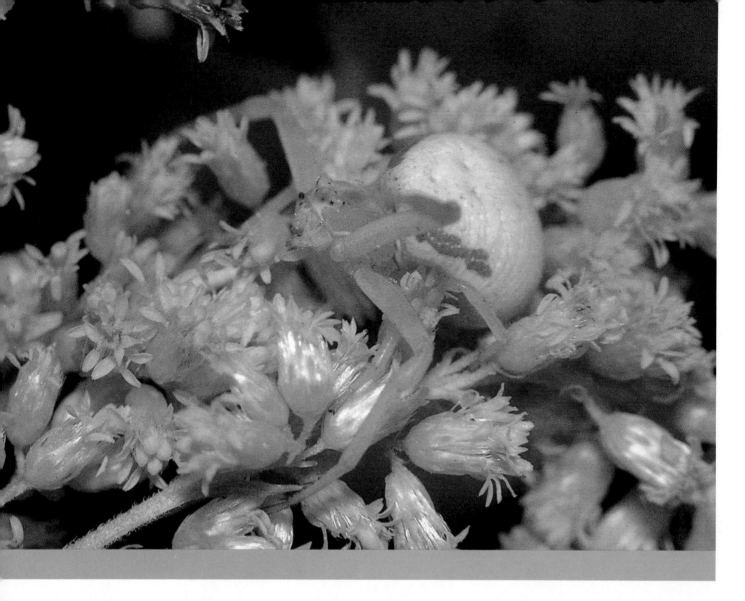

The Perception of Polarized Light

Both hunting spiders and weavers use the perception of polarized light to orient themselves. In spiders with both main and secondary eyes, the retinas of the main eyes have two functions: image formation as well as the perception of polarized light. The top section of the retina forms the image while the bottom detects the path of the light rays.

Bees and cephalopods use their knowledge of the path of light rays to navigate in overcast weather or in the depths of the sea where the overall glare makes light appear to ordinary eyes to come from all directions. One doesn't think of the hunting spider's movements through flowers and leaves as coming under the heading of nav-igation, but with the limited focal length of their lenses, we can think of their image-forming eyes as macro telephoto lenses—everything else is out of focus.

Color Vision in Spiders

It is now apparent that jumping spiders do possess a limited form of color vision. Their rhabdoms are located at several different layers, each of which is sensitive to a different wavelength. Their visual pigment peaks in the ultraviolet as well as the green area of the spectrum, and their ultraviolet markings are probably visible to other members of this species. Color vision in other spiders is much more limited, and according to most experts has reached only the level

▲

Color vision is not widespread among spiders; however, the crab spider (**Misumena vatia**) *can change color from white to yellow or vice versa to camouflage it from its prey.*

of fish and some birds in members of the salticids, or jumpers.

One of the few other spiders to have any possibility of color vision is the crab spider, *Misumena vatia*. Like the jumping spider, it has main eyes, but it can also change color from yellow to white. The crab spider hides in wait and ambushes insects, such as flies, bees and butterflies. On its back is a large red marking that is probably invisible to most insects with vision in the ultraviolet. It is generally believed to be a warning sign to birds, who can see it, that this particular creature is noxious.

4 Insects

It is to insects that we owe the wide variety of colors in flowering plants. Insects, after all, are the pollinators of the plant world. Without them, plants would neither flower nor bear fruit. Flowering plants and winged insects evolved at the same time in the earth's history. The first pollinators were the beetles, and they still pollinate the more primitive flowers, such as laurel, magnolias and water lillies; but only the long-tongued, winged insects can reach the pollen in the fused tubes of the more advanced plants.

But the attraction is not limited to color; there are some plants, like the bee orchid, for example, that mimic an insect's appearance so well that the insect actually attempts to copulate with it, spreading pollen in the process. If the bee's vision were poor, nature would not have had to invent such an elaborate subterfuge. We know now that insects see far better than most of us have been led to believe. In fact, nature has created quite a few flowers whose appearance mimics that of specific insects; the danger, however, is that if the pollinating insect dies out, the plant also becomes extinct.

Older vision theory was of the opinion that the eye of the insect was best adapted for detecting movement but permitted only a coarse image of the world. That view is now being challenged. It is likely that the visual range of the insect eye is limited to objects that are fairly close by human standards but that within that range some insects can distinguish fine detail. Contemporary vision scientists such as Kirschfield, a prominent researcher in this field, are convinced

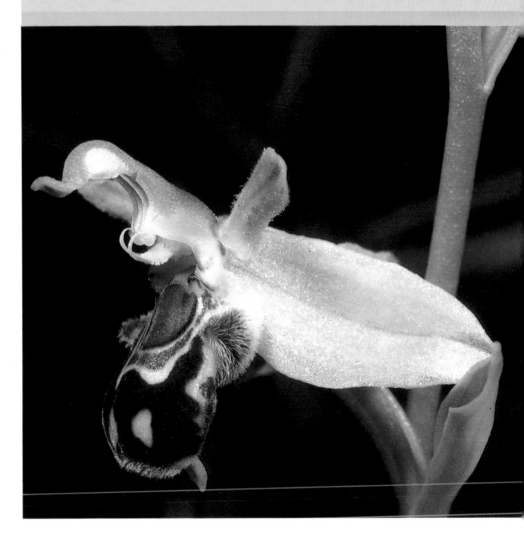

that it is the size of the photoreceptors and not the lens system that determines the clarity of what insects see. The bee's photoreceptors, for example, are about the same size as our own. Also, Kirschfield has examined the brain of the fly and found that the number of neurons devoted to visual points far exceeds the number of human visual connections. One thing is sure—the spectrum of colors seen by insects is wider than our own;

▲

The bee orchid. Flowering plants and winged insects developed at the same time, and their interdependence is most obvious in plants that actually mimic a specific insect's appearance in order to attract them for pollination.

it ranges from ultraviolet into the near infrared in the case of some butterflies, while the human spectrum is limited to violet through red.

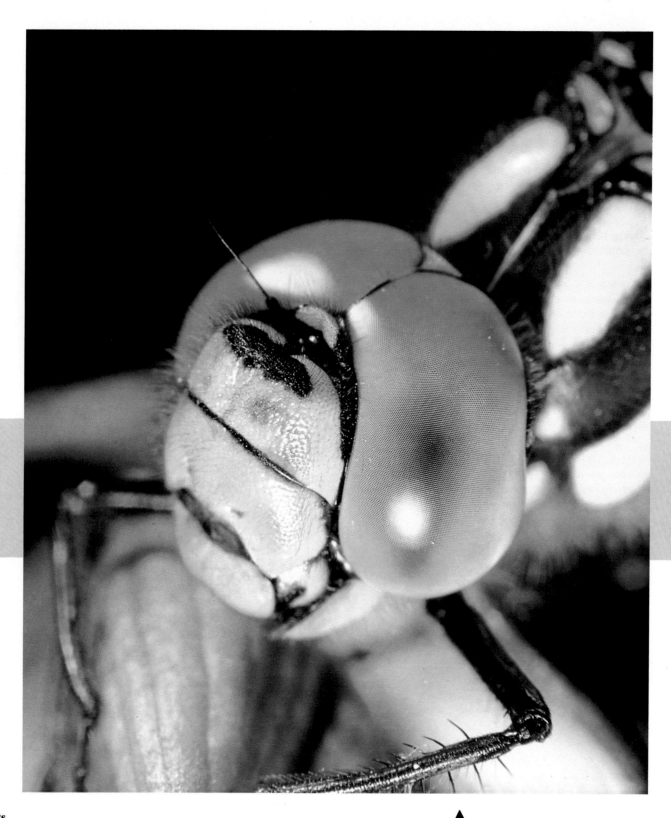

▲

Southern aeshna dragonfly. The compound eyes of the dragonfly have more facets than any other insect, numbering from 28,000 to about 30,000 lenslets in each eye.

The Compound Eye

It is the lens system of the insect eye, known as the compound eye, that differs so greatly from that of the vertebrate eye. While some insects have additional simple eyes, these have no power of image formation and are limited to faint discrimination of movement and perhaps some color. In some winged insects, the simple eyes may have important navigational functions, maintaining the insects' position relative to the horizon. But it is the compound eye that is the basic eye of the insect world.

For years, science-fiction films have shown what purports to be the insect's view of the world—the same image repeated over and over again. The reality is much more intriguing. In the compound eye, the lens is divided into separate facets and individual refracting units called ommatidia; sometimes there are thousands of them in each eye. Lens and cornea are one, in contrast to the vertebrate eye. And the image transmitted by each small lens is not the same overall picture but only the small portion of the visual field that is within its angular range. The separate parts of the field are transmitted to the photoreceptors of the ommatidia, and it is here that the overall image is fused.

The number of these facets in the compound eye varies considerably from insect to insect. The dragonfly leads with 28,000 to 30,000; it's enormous eyes produce an almost-hemispherical view of the world. In contrast, the dark-adapted eye of the underground worker ant, *Solenopsis,* has only nine facets per eye. Worker and drone bees have many more facets than the queen (who is limited to only 3,000 to 4,000), since those who do not forage for their food need not see as well. City-dwellers who have suffered the ravages of the cockroach *Periplaneta americana* may be interested to know that that insect seeks your crumbs with eyes consisting of 2,000 facets each.

The facets of the compound eye can also vary in shape. Where there are few facets they tend to be round, but when they are more numerous and packed tightly together, their shape becomes hexagonal.

In addition, the facets can vary in size, even in the same eye. For example, the facets in the center of the bee's eye are larger (22nm in diameter) than at the top (17nm in diameter): The bee is obviously more concerned about what it sees dead ahead. However, the facets on the top of the

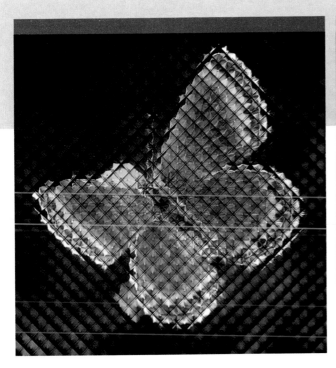

▲
Vision scientists used to think that the vision of most insects resembles a coarse mosaic, but this is more likely true of insects with few lenslets and less numerous photoreceptors.

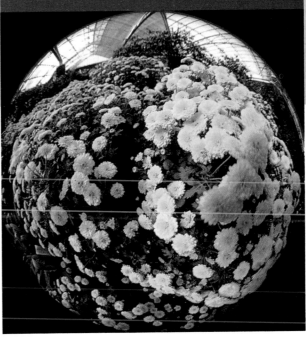

▲
A number of modern vision theorists believe that the visual image is fused at the level of the photoreceptors, and since bees and dragonflies have as many photoreceptors per square millimeter as the human eye, their images, close up, should be as good or better than our own.

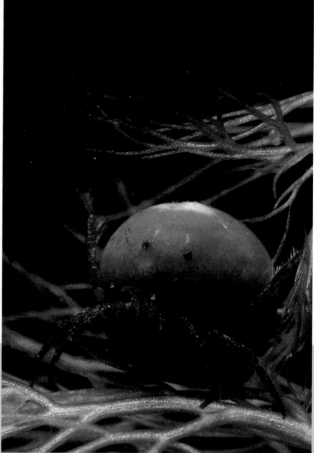

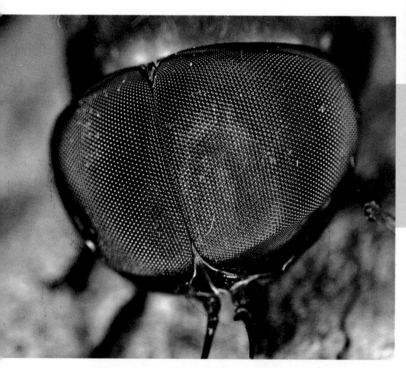

dragonfly eye are twice the size of those on the bottom.

Light is transmitted from each lens by a crystalline cone that functions as a light guide. At the base of the cone are radially arranged nerve cells, or rhabdomeres, which contain the individual photoreceptors called rhabdoms. The combination of lens facet, crystalline cone and rhabdomere makes up the basic refracting (light-bending) facet known as the ommatidium.

The Optics of the Compound Eye

It is a scientific rule of thumb that the larger the eye, the better its resolving power, or acuity. To resolve light means to be able to see changes in brightness at microscopic levels. Kirschfield estimates that the compound eye would have to be at least one meter in diameter to match the overall resolving power of the human eye. What heavy heads we would have to support!

Without question, the compound eye is the eye of smaller creatures (the lobster's compound eye is the largest). But perhaps it is just nature's way of providing a creature with an optical mechanism that suits its own needs: The insect has no need to see clearly at a great distance, but some can distinguish fine detail close up. For example, *Colias,* a butterfly, can distinguish two points separated by as little as 30 microns, while the human eye has a minimum distinguishable distance of 100 microns. To appreciate this, imagine the fine detail of a flower or twig that escapes our own eyes. It all depends on one's point of view.

The compound eye is a fixed-focus eye; there is no accommodation for near and far vision. If an insect wants to see an object better, it must move closer; but unlike the vertebrate eye, it is completely free of both the color distortion and the spherical aberration that plague the larger vertebrate eye. Each lens facet transmits light to its own photoreceptors or those that are close by, so that the eye gets an equally sharp picture from all directions. By contrast, the vertebrate eye has high resolution only in the area of greatest photoreceptor concentration (the fovea in our case); the greater the distance from the fovea, the greater the visual aberrations.

We are largely unaware of this phenomenon because our eyes are constantly shifting. But the area we see clearly at any given time is no larger than the tip of our thumb, and if you will concentrate your vision on a word in the center of this page, you will become aware of the lack of clarity in the area around it.

Like all invertebrate photoreceptors, the rhabdoms face toward the lens and the incoming light. The number of rhabdoms in each ommatidium varies according to species. For example, the common house fly has eight in each ommatidium, but it has many thousands of ommatidia in each eye.

One of the problems that nature faces over and over again is accommodating an eye for vision at night. There are both diurnal and nocturnal forms of the compound eye. As in the vertebrate eye, nature has had to make a compromise: Generally, acuity is sacrificed for sensitivity. The two types of compound eye are known as the apposition eye and the superposition eye, and they differ from one another primarily in the way that light is transmitted to the rhabdoms.

Like many other insects, the harlequin beetle's eyes curve around its antennae, giving it an unusual field of vision.

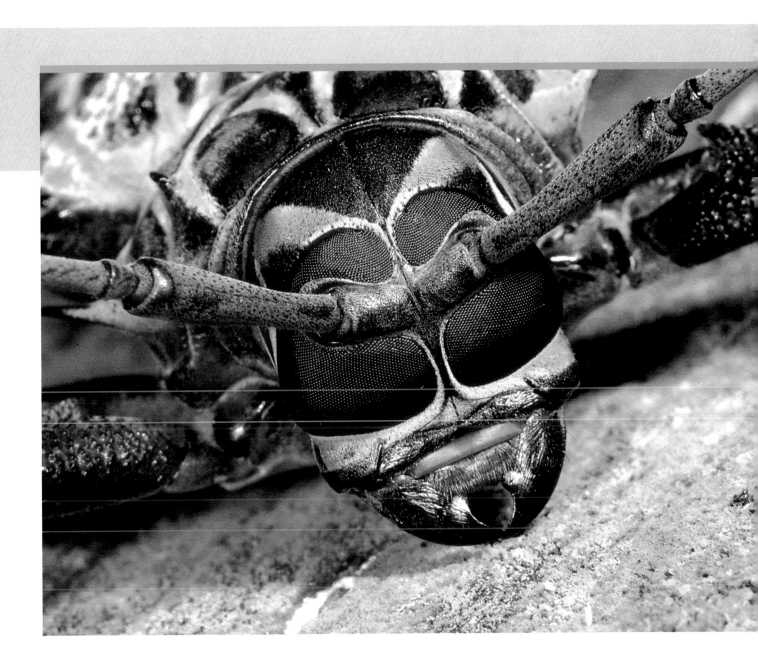

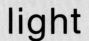

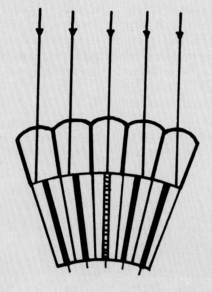
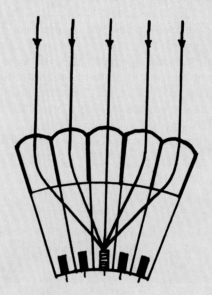

The Apposition Eye

The apposition compound eye, found in diurnal insects, gives the sharper image of the two. Diurnal insects are mainly land-dwelling or shore-dwelling, like the damselfly and all forms of flies and even mosquitoes.

The reason for the sharpness of the apposition eye's image is that light from only its own lens facet reaches the rhabdoms of each ommatidium. The crystalline cone, which acts as a light guide, is completely surrounded by screening pigment that absorbs any stray light from nearby facets. This results in a very small lens aperture for each facet and thus the sharpness of the image formed. The focal length of each lens is equal to or slightly longer than the crystalline cone, so that the beams of light entering the cylinder converge at the end of the cone on the waiting rhabdoms, which means that the image formed on the rhabdoms is upside down.

The pupillary apertures of animals' eyes are frequently compared to the f-stop of a camera lens. An f-stop can be defined as the focal length of a lens—the maximum distance over which it can form an image—divided by the aperture. Animals that must see bright points of light against dark backgrounds (dim light), and this includes the majority of nocturnal animals, have evolved large apertures and small f-stops. While our own eyes open as wide as 7 or 8mm, the best resolution of the human eye occurs at 2.4mm. Strangely, this matches that of the bee, even though the ratio of pupillary area in man to bee is 10^5:1. But both the ratio of focal length to aperture and the size of photoreceptors are the same despite the enormous difference in the size of the bee eye and that of the human. We know that a camera lens can shoot at low light levels when it has an f-stop of f1.4. But the f-stops of nocturnal insects are much lower; the flour moth, *Ephestia*, has an f-stop of 1.2mm, which means its eyes can form an image at much lower light levels, where the bee would be virtually blind.

▲

Apposition and superposition eyes. Apposition eyes create a very clear image because the light from each ommatidium is contained and falls only on its own photoreceptors (rhabdoms), while the superposition eye permits light from adjacent ommatidia to fall on other rhabdoms, increasing the chances of light absorption but degrading the quality of the image.

The Superposition Eye

This eye is also called the clear-zone eye because of the additional crystalline tract that separates the crystalline cone from the lens. As the word *crystalline* implies, light can pass through the tract. Consequently, light passing through the lens facets of this eye must travel a greater distance before reaching the rhabdoms. The cone is about twice the focal length of the lens, so that parallel beams of light entering the cone intersect and then repeat their paths in reverse. Thus the image received by the rhabdoms in the supposition eye is right-side-up (in contrast to images received both by the apposition eye and the vertebrate eye), and thus the nocturnal insect's brain does not have to compensate.

Unlike the apposition eye, however, the crystalline cone of the superposition eye is not always completely surrounded by screening pigment absorbing stray light. Superposition eyes have two states: a dark-adapted state in which the screening pigment moves away from the crystalline cone and rhabdomeres, leaving them exposed to light from other ommatidia; and a light-adapted state, in which the pigment moves back to cover. The acuity of the nocturnal insect's eye is best during the light-adapted state since acuity is increased when the integrity of the ommatidium is maintained. However, since nocturnal insects must gather all available light in order to see in the dark, the pooling of light that takes place when screening pigment has receded takes precedence.

Unlike the apposition eye,

which forms its individual images side by side, the superposition eye's images are formed on top of each other. Since the oblique rays from neighboring images blur the image formed by each facet, the price paid for the increased sensitivity is lack of clarity, though there is considerable variation in the quality of vision in nocturnal insects. Large moths and the nocturnal butterfly *Toxidia* have excellent vision, but they are exceptions to the rule.

Besides nocturnal insects, the superposition eye is found in aquatic insects and those that live underground or in dim light.

At the beginning of this project I wondered how other creatures viewed objects like flowers, trees or stars. I am not alone in my curiosity. Kirschfield believes that while stars are invisible to diurnal insects, the evening star, Venus, can be seen by the flour moth, *Ephestia*. Remember that *Ephestia* has an f-stop of 1.2mm. Even though its individual lens facets are minute in comparison with the

human lens, their images are superimposed upon one another at the photoreceptor level, which significantly increases the effective apperture of the eye. Also, the size of the rhabdomic photoreceptors in *Ephestia* are considerably larger, about 20 microns, than those of the bee, which are only 1 micron or 2 microns in diameter. Thus they absorb more light at night.

Problems of the Compound Lens

Why can't *Ephestia* see more distant stars? One of the drawbacks of the compound lens has to do with the optical phenomenom of diffraction. Remember that as photons move through space, they are vibrating at incredible speed. Sometimes when they pass through a very small opening, such as the minute lens facets of the insect eye, the vibrating photon catches or kicks off the edge of the lens. As a result, the photon does not land in one point but in a series of alternating light and dark concentric circles known as an Airy pattern. It is the diameter of the Airy pattern that limits the resolution of the compound eye. According to Kirschfield, it requires at least 5 photoreceptors to scan the diameter of the Airy discs and 20 to scan the entire area. This limits the resolution powers of the compound eye. Add to this the lack of available light at night and you have the answer.

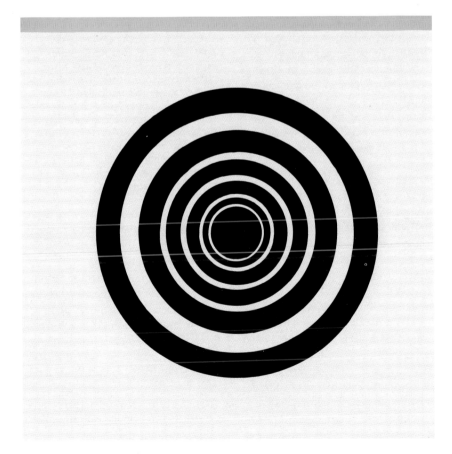

◄

The Airy disc. One of the reasons for the inability of insects to see stars is the minute size of the individual lenslets of their eyes. Photons of light hit against the side of the lens as they enter the eye, so that the visual information does not form a point but instead a series of darker and lighter concentric circles that may be too large for individual photoreceptors to absorb. Thus, small points of light at great distances are invisible, although the flour moth, **Ephestia,** *may be able to see Venus, the evening star.*

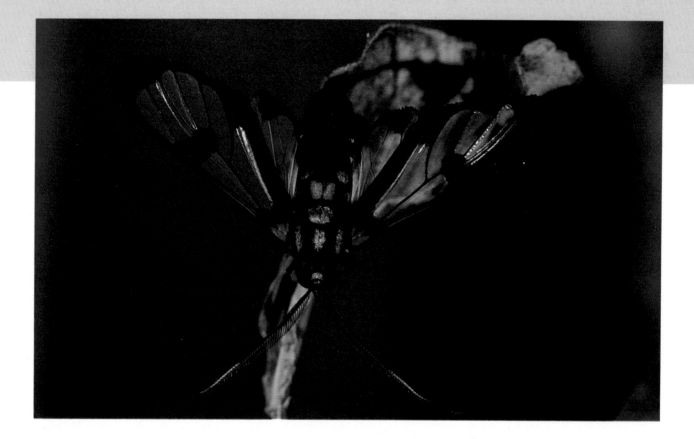

The Photoreceptors of the Compound Eye

Generally, rhabdoms are far longer than the corresponding rods and cones in the vertebrate eye. The rhabdoms themselves are composed of layers of tiny cells called microvilli on which are suspended molecules of visual pigment. The rhabdoms extend the length of the elongated rhabdomere, or retinula cell, as it is also called. However, rhabdoms contain much less visual pigment than do vertebrate photoreceptors.

One of the reasons for the decreased amount of pigment may be that in invertebrates, after they have absorbed a photon of light the chromoproteins of visual pigment do not immediately fall apart as they do in the vertebrate eye. Instead they are altered to form another type of rhodopsin, called metarhodopsin, which can still absorb photons but in a range limited to 450nm through 500nm (that's the blue and blue-green area of the spectrum). After the metarho-

dopsin molecule absorbs a photon, however, it does fall apart and must reconstitute itself with Vitamin A_1, though this process occurs more rapidly than in the vertebrate eye.

Images take place in time as well as space. One of the reasons that modern vision theory believes insect vision superior to what had been thought previously is that visual acuity is also dependent on the speed with which images can be formed on the photoreceptors. We know that in vertebrates it takes longer for the dark-adapted eye to form an image than the light-adapted eye. But some insect eyes perceive many more images per second than do human eyes. The flicker-fusion cycle of our eyes is measured at 50 to 60 per second in bright light and 10 per second in dim light. But the flicker-fusion cycle for winged insects can be as high as 300 per second (crickets are lower with only 45 per second). A movie passing before the eyes of a winged insect at 24 frames per second may look like a series of still photographs. The images that pass before the human eye

▲

Comet tail moth (right) and an Amazonian moth of the family Ctenuchidae. Moths are rare among nocturnal creatures in having color vision. They may even be able to see colors at night when our own vision has become monochromatic. Moths use moonlight and starlight as a guide to maintaining a specific angle during flight, but in the presence of a lamp or flame this behavior leads to their doom as they continuously circle, getting closer and closer to the heat that ultimately destroys them.

move at a far more leisurely pace yet, after all, we have no need to catch our prey on the fly.

Winged insects have the best overall vision in the insect kingdom. The reason for this superiority is that these insects have tiers of photoreceptors arranged in single layers. Each facet of a dragonfly eye, for example, has eight retinula cells ordered in four layers. Similarly, damselflies have three tiers of receptors in each facet. The cells fuse, creating an especially long rhabdom capable of a high percentage of light absorption.

Tapetum and Iridescence in the Insect Eye

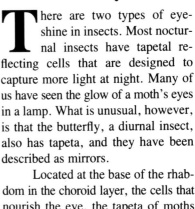

There are two types of eyeshine in insects. Most nocturnal insects have tapetal reflecting cells that are designed to capture more light at night. Many of us have seen the glow of a moth's eyes in a lamp. What is unusual, however, is that the butterfly, a diurnal insect, also has tapeta, and they have been described as mirrors.

Located at the base of the rhabdom in the choroid layer, the cells that nourish the eye, the tapeta of moths are made up of densely packed tubes filled with air (tracheole bushes). Each tracheole is separated from its neighbors by another pocket of air, but the butterflies' tapeta are made up of cytoplasmic plates that alternate with air spaces. The tapeta of butterflies are more like interference filters. Wavelengths of light that are rejected by the filter are reflected back by the mirrorlike cells. Those that are acceptable pass. What is unusual in butterflies is that each mirror system can be completely different from its neighboring rhabdomes. Thus there can be a wide variety in the color of their tapetal reflections. Perhaps the tapeta of butterflies help extend the color vision of these insects into the evening. While color vision is rare in most nocturnal creatures, it is known to exist in a variety of moths, who see in color even when we would be color blind. The light reflected by tapetal cells in the upper regions of the eyes of butterflies and moths is primarily shortwave; that reflected by the lower portion has a long wavelength.

Iridescent Corneas

Iridescent corneas are a widespread phenomenon in the insect world. Certainly iridescent corneas act as interference filters, reinforcing some wavelengths of light and canceling others. They may help the insect by reinforcing only those wavelengths of light to which its photoreceptors are most sensitive.

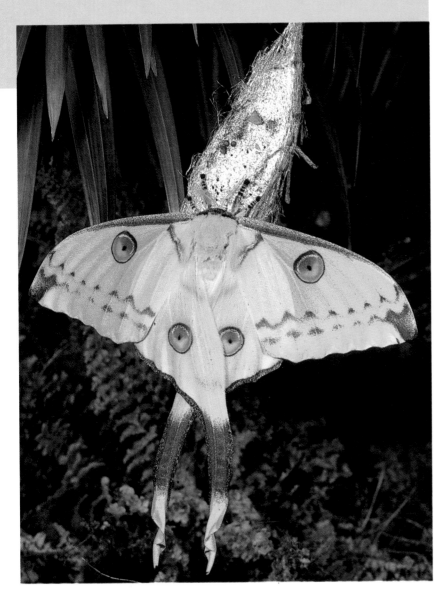

The Perception of Polarized Light

No matter what the weather, many insects know the position of the sun. Since the microvilli within the rhabdoms (the cells from which visual pigment is suspended) are arranged at right angles to one another, the visual pigment is able to detect the direction from which the light comes.

This perception of the plane of polarized light is a distinct aid to navigation. Moreover, bees can maintain the sun as their fixed point of reference, even taking into account the movement of the sun across the sky. Not only can they perceive polarized light, but bees use a visual code to show other bees the way to food through the performance of complex movements that its decipherer, Friederick Von Frisch, calls a "dance." The angle of the dance in relation to the sun indicates the food's direction; the speed of the movements, the distance. By performing the dance themselves, the other bees memorize the directions. This is the most complex behavior in the insect world based on visual perception.

More primitive insects cannot detect polarized light because the arrangement of their microvilli is haphazard. Higher orders of insects, like all other creatures, tend to greater organization of the visual mechanisms.

Visual Tracking by the Winged Insect

For insects as well as birds, the requirements of flying, landing and catching prey in mid-flight demand great visual acuity. Creatures like ourselves, who move their eyes in their sockets, use their interocular muscles (there are six in the human eye) to maintain a steady image on the retina while turning their bodies. But the insect's eyes are immobile, and in order for them to follow a moving object, they must turn their entire bodies, no mean feat for a creature whose soft body parts (head, thorax and abdomen) are enclosed in a hard exterior skeleton.

But winged insects, the most advanced members of the insect world, do have some visual assets. Remember that their eyes process many, many more images per second than our own. (If you've ever seen a high-speed film, you know the detail missed by our own eyes.) Also, the total image in their entire visual field is in focus, in contrast to our own limited foveal area. Their eyes are free of astigmatism and color aberration. There is also the size and placement of their eyes.

Dragonflies and members of the fly family have the largest eyes in the insect world. The eyes of the dragonfly are so large that it has an almost hemispherical view of the world. The eyes of the fly are at the ends of long protuberances with such a great distance between each eye that the visual base exceeds the width of its body. Like an optical telemeter, the fly is able to estimate distance with incredible accuracy by focusing on an object and comparing the angle from each eye. By the way, we do this ourselves though we are not consciously aware of it. Our brain is constantly comparing the differences between the angle from each eye to the sighted object, using feedback from the eye muscles. This is what allows a baseball pitcher to put a ball over the plate with such accuracy.

Motion is of the utmost importance to the sharpness of insect vision, as it is to our own. One of the reasons is that once visual pigment has decomposed, it needs time to reconstitute itself, granted that the metarhodopsin stage makes the process quicker in invertebrates. Fortunately, most creatures have millions of photoreceptors. When an image moves relative to the eye, because the object has moved or the eye has moved, or both, the moving image triggers new photoreceptors and allows the cells that were stimulated originally to recover. Most vertebrate eyes make constant small jumps, or saccades as they are called, that change the photoreceptors responding to the image. While insect eyes themselves are immobile, the insect is usually in motion, particularly the winged insect. Also, insect bodies quiver constantly due to heart and respiratory movements.

▼

Diopsis has eyes perched on the ends of stalks, an unusual arrangement for flying insects but quite common in crustaceans that also have compound eyes.

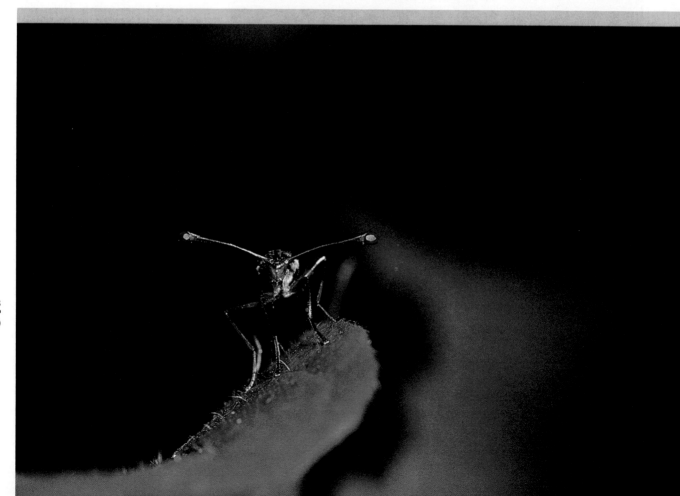

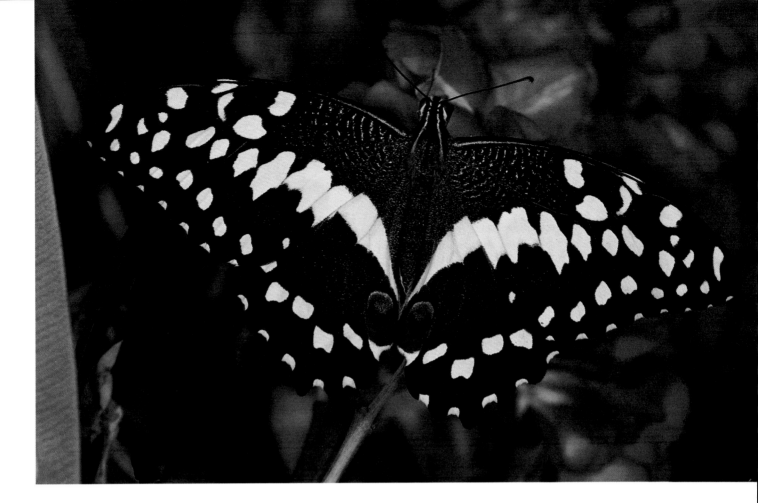

Registering motion visually consists of tracking the object by following it with the eyes or letting it pass over the photoreceptors. Larger lens facets within the insect eye indicate areas of increased sensitivity to images that pass over that area. Wide angles between facets are also a sign. Fast-flying and jumping insects have wider horizontal than vertical visual angles, which indicates a sensitivity to objects that pass across the visual field rather than up and down. The rhabdoms of more advanced insects are also more specialized; for example, those of the hover fly, *Syritta*, will fire only if the passing object falls within a certain size range. But some rhabdoms can adjust their size preference depending on the speed of the image. This means that they recognize the characteristics of other creatures by their size and speed.

This behavior is probably programmed into the insect eye rather than being a conscious decision of the insect brain. Again, one is made aware of the sophistication of the eye, not only as an instrument of vision but as an organ capable of responding to complex situations without recourse to the brain.

Animals have various methods of compensating to hold some part of the visual field steady while they themselves move. Flying insects make deliberate jumps in flight to mitigate their involuntary movements caused by drafts or the quivering of their own bodies: It is easier to prepare the eyes for one's own movements than to be caught unawares. Since the fly's greatest acuity is to images in front of it, it keeps its eyes fixed on an object a few inches away; anything in between is out of focus, but at least that part of the visual field is stable. Compensation for movement is not found only among insects. Birds first push their head forward and then keep it still as the body catches up. The dogfish shark fixes its eyes on an area about three feet away and counterrotates the eyes as it swims from side to side. In effect, mammalian saccades enable selected areas of the vi-

▲

Butterflies probably have the widest spectrum of color vision in the insect world, going beyond that of the bee, which we know is trichromatic. Some butterflies may even have a fourth color receptor, allowing them to see longer wavelengths of light as well as the very short ultraviolet wavelengths.

sual field to be constantly within the view of the highest area of photoreceptor concentration.

It has been suggested that one of the reasons flying insects have acquired relatively advanced color vision is that color is one feature that can be recognized independently of background. Even if an object is blurred, it is possible to determine its color. Butterflies, in particular, respond to color; the *Morpho* butterfly always flies to blue lures, while other species show an increased response to red. This is in contrast to the response of certain highly developed vertebrates, such as cats, who appear to respond more to shape than to color.

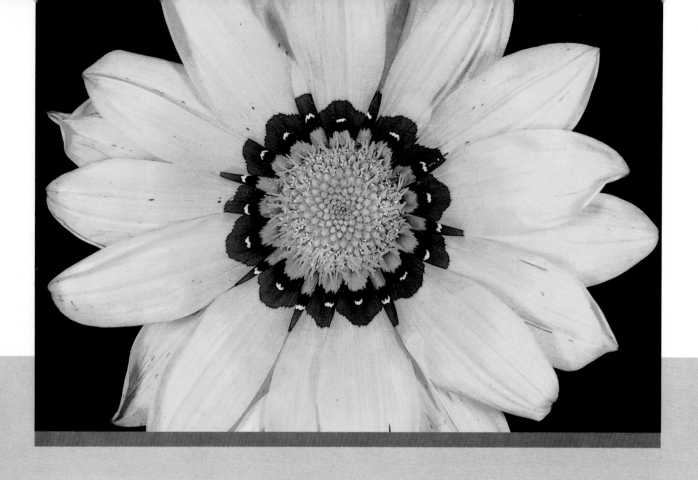

Color Vision in Insects

Color vision is the rule rather than the exception in the insect world. It extends even to nocturnal insects, though color vision among nocturnal animals is rare indeed. Moths are known to have some color vision, which the distinguished Russian entomologist, Morzhokin-Porschnyakov, attributes to their need for protective coloration during the day. A diurnal butterfly, *Deilephila livornica,* can recognize colors in faint twilight, which is beyond the color perceptions of man. Our own vision is largely monochromatic in low light.

Until recently, most of the research on insects consisted of testing behavior or was limited to the photoreceptor level. Now researchers have begun to investigate the neural mechanisms devoted to vision, a daunting task given the smallness of these creatures' eyes. The Electrophysiological techniques are permitting vision science to explore the more complex interactions that occur as information is transmitted to the brain.

Theories of color are being explored that, if correct, would indicate that insects' color perceptions differ markedly from our own. But first, what do we know from behavioral experiments and the nature of photoreceptors?

Most insects have only two types of visual pigment. (Each ommatidium is limited to one type of pigment.) This means that its color range is limited but that within that range it may be able to distinguish between hues that to the human eye appear the same. The housefly can distinguish colors separated by as little as 3nm to 7nm in the area of the spectrum to which it is most sensitive. Other insects are limited to longer wavelengths and cannot distinguish blues, violets and ultraviolets. The dragonfly is supposedly one such example.

The widest range of color vision among insects belongs to bees and butterflies. The bee, like ourselves, is trichromatic; that is, its photoreceptors contain three types of visual pigment, though its sensitivity is shifted toward the ultraviolet end of the spectrum and excludes longer wavelengths in the red area. The ability to test visual pigment and find its exact peak wavelength sensitivity has been an enormous advantage to science in deciphering other creatures' color ranges. We also know that the best color vision occurs in the area where the spectral sensitivities of two pigments overlap, and in the case of trichromats there are two overlap areas instead of one.

The bee's color sensitivity begins at about 345nm and extends to 550nm. According to Autrum, a well-known German vision scientist, its best color discrimination occurs between 480nm and 510nm in the blue area of the spectrum. Here, color changes rapidly with wavelength. While bees have been known to alight on red California poppies, for exam-

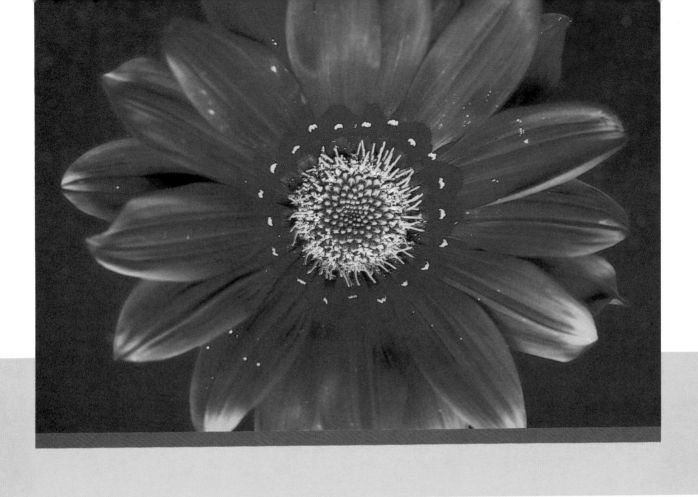

▲ ▲

Ganzania daisies as they appear to us and to insects whose color vision extends into the ultraviolet area of the spectrum. Markings invisible to our eyes show insects the way to the pollen, like landing lights at an airport. Similarly, insects that appear dull to us are visibly different to their species mates and other insects with ultraviolet vision.

ple, they may see them only as dark spots against a green background. But the petals of the poppies may also reflect ultraviolet light, to which the bee's eyes are sensitive. In fact, a flower that appears white to us may actually reflect ultraviolet light and thus appear colored to the bee. The primary colors of the bee also differ from our own (red, green and blue) and instead fall in the blue, yellow and ultraviolet areas of the spectrum. After yellow, instead of seeing oranges and reds, the bee may see what is called "bee purple."

Butterflies are such beautifully patterned and colors creatures that one would expect them to have a wide color range, and they do. Until recently it was thought that bees had the widest color vision, but some butterflies may even have a fourth visual pigment. There are butterflies with acute sensitivity to ultraviolet. To the human eye, for instance, the male and female *Colias* appear virtually identical, but when they are photographed under ultraviolet light, there is a remarkable difference in their coloring and patterns.

Other butterflies show a distinct preference for red: *Heliconius erato, Papilio troilus* and *Colias eurthemus* are some examples. In fact, some butterflies and fireflies have wavelength sensitivities that go as high as 690nm, in the near infrared. However, *Heliconius erato's* response to red is merely romantic; it responds to red during courtship but to yellow for food. Brightness values also change from species to species in butterflies;

supposedly all butterflies see yellow brightly, though red and orange appear dark to *Satyridae* and light to *Nymphalidae, Pieridae* and *Lycaenidae*.

A French vision scientist, Pierre Caricaburru, has advanced a theory of color vision among insects that indicates a dramatic color shift. We know that color shifts occur in other creatures; cyprihid fish, including members of the goldfish family, have color vision that is shifted to longer wavelengths; what we see as yellow, they see more as orange. Caricaburru's theories suggest a color shift that is complicated by the presence of ultraviolet sensitivity. Color changes are quite dramatic: What we see as blue is perceived as green or cyan; green becomes red or magenta, and red becomes blue or white, just to give a few examples.

Pierre Caricaburru has used photographic experiments to give what he calls an "intuitive" sense of the insect's color vision. Photographing

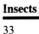

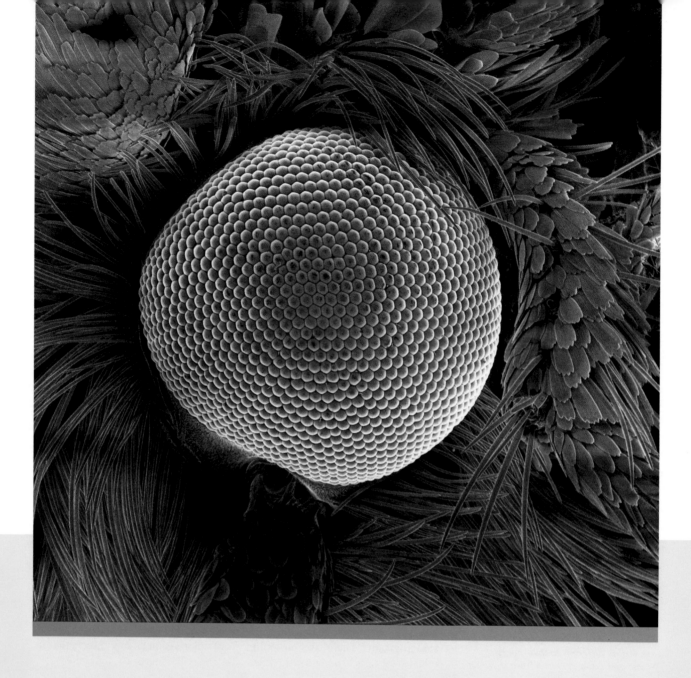

human skin and plants with a variety
of filters, including one ultraviolet
filter, and using a special printing
method, he feels that he has successfully shown how insects see color.
Alpine skin becomes brown; a magenta anemone is seen as cyan, yet a
red anemone is seen as black. Is it
possible that insects fly through a
world of red leaves and green sky,
that a green apple looks the same to
an insect as a yellow lemon?

Although not accepted by the

entire scientific world, theories of
color shift are also being explored by
other researchers, Swihart of the
University of Tampa and Gordon of
the University of South Florida believe that opponent color mechanisms in the insect brain alter the
transmission of the color message so
that the type of visual pigment found
in the insect photoreceptor is only part
of the story. In their examination of
the receptors in butterflies, they believe they have found a blue/orange

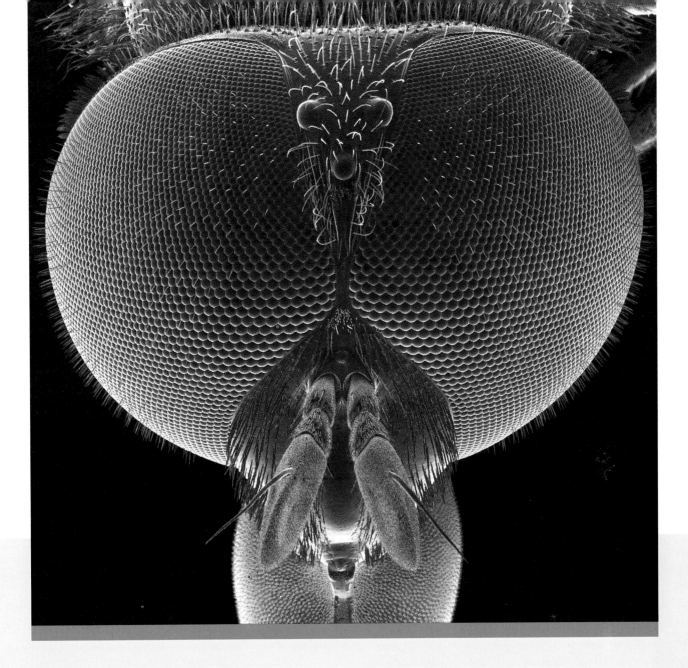

fiber whose integrating activity may preclude an insect's ability to see the color green. Again, this is theory and not accepted scientific fact, but it does indicate the areas that are being explored by vision scientists.

Glare Reduction in Insects

Since insects have no eyelids, glare reduction is important to many insects with large com-pound eyes, and nature has provided them with a number of devices to decrease the reflection of light on the surface and increase the transparency of the corneal lenses. This is particularly true for insects with four membranous wings, such as ant lions or doodlebugs. Small conical nipples visible to the human eye only with a microscope appear on the axes of the ommatidia in a hexagonal pattern and function as an anti-glare device. This is particularly true of moths, which also need to reduce the reflection of their eyes during the day.

But winged insects have a special problem with their large eyes, some of which are almost spherical. Some lenses are always facing the sun, which is most destructive to their vulnerable photoreceptors. Such insects have what has been described as longitudinal pupils, screening pigment-containing granules that move swiftly back and forth to protect the rhabdoms.

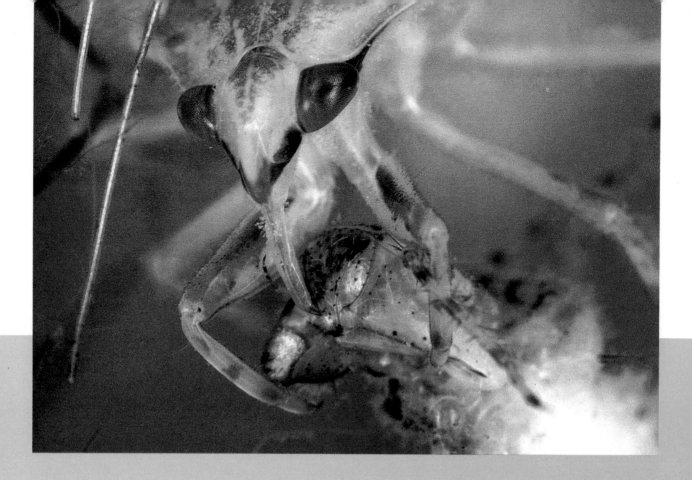

Aquatic Insects

While terrestrial insects' lenses are convex, the lenses of many aquatic insects are flat. Since the refracting index of flat lenses changes less than that of convex lenses when the insect goes from one medium to another, the insect's vision remains relatively constant when it passes from air to water or vice versa. Our own lenses are convex, so that when we swim under water, a fairly rare occurrence for most of us, we become farsighted without the use of goggles or a mask. But the human eye has a wide range of vision, and the insect is far more limited. A flat lens, therefore, ensures a more constant focal length for a creature that moves constantly between air and water to find food.

This holds true mainly for insects with hard lenses. When the lenses are made of soft, vitreous substance, they are spherical in shape. These are called pseudocone or acone ommatidia.

When the beetle *Gyrinus* swims across the surface of the water, its dorsal eyes remain above the surface looking over the pond, while the ventral eyes see below the surface. The structure of each set of eyes matches the environment in which they function. The dorsal eyes are apposition eyes and the underwater eyes are supposition eyes.

Variations in the Insect Compound Eye

While most insects have either apposition eyes or superposition eyes, there are a few exceptions. The praying mantis forms supposition images in the back facets of its eyes while the frontal ommatidia form the more acute apposition images. Acuity may be more important here since the frontal images also give the insect visual overlap and depth perception. The male *Cleonus* forms superposition

▲

The pond vampire water bug has fiery red eyes. The lenses of most aquatic insects are flat so that the refraction between air and water remains relatively constant.

images on the upper part of its eye and apposition images on the lower. Insects with both types of image-creating mechanisms have the advantage that they can function in both bright and dim light.

Other variations concern color perception. Some insects have color vision in only a part of their eyes. *Libellula* and *Callipadra* see color only in the upper half of the eye, while the cockroach and dragonfly see color in only the lower portion. The dragonfly hunts while flying and may not need color vision to spot its prey's silhouette against the sky, but color vision in the lower portion of the eye may give it the increased contrast sensitivity it needs to find food against the more varied terrestrial background.

Conclusion

The optic lobes of the insect are the most highly developed areas of its brain. Despite these creatures' small size, the visual connecting links of some of the winged insects are more numerous than our own, and the bee's rhabdoms are the same size as our own rods and cones. Vision science appears to be moving away from the belief that the insect sees simply a coarse mosaic of the world; in the case of higher winged insects that may not be true. That the winged insect's eyes are superior to ours at detecting motion is without question.

In behavioral tests, bees have shown that they can distinguish shapes such as circles, ellipses and triangles. But the movements of the bee's food dance already exhibits a level of sophisticated abstraction in a very tiny brain.

All eyes are scanning or sampling devices. The eyes of insects sample a world that is much smaller and closer to themselves. Theirs is a small eye in a tiny body. Undoubtedly the compound eye is the eye of smaller creatures, even though the earliest dragonflies had a wingspan of 2 feet and obviously a much larger eye. Theirs is a world of twigs, leaves and flowers. They have no need to separate the forest from the trees.

But there is no denying the extraordinary range of their color vision, particularly that of bees and, even more so, butterflies. Winged insects more than other creatures seem to have escaped the effects of early evolution in the seas, which blocked all ultraviolet light. Not so their close relations the crustaceans, whose color visual experience is far more limited despite a very similar eye.

▼

The glowworm can create its own light to attract mates. Unlike the light we create with fire or electricity, bioluminescent light is called cold light, giving off far more light than heat.

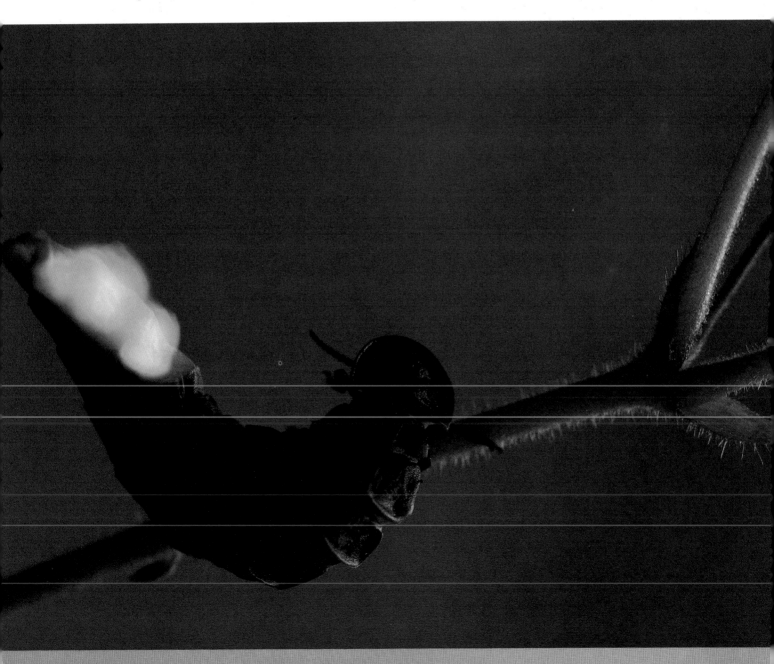

5 *Crustaceans*

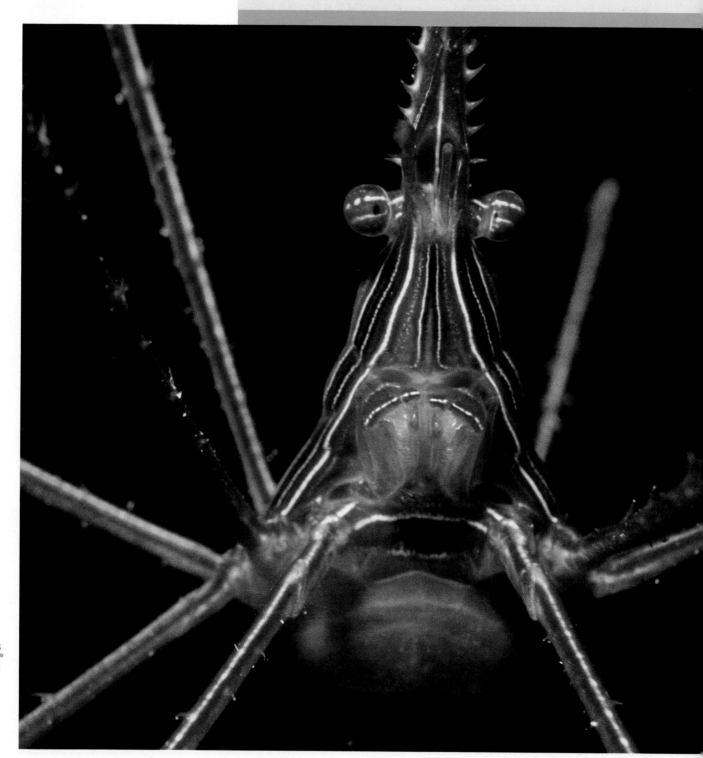

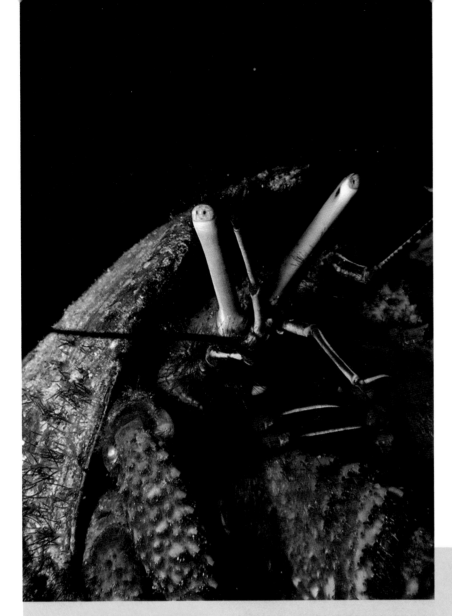

Like spiders and scorpions, crustaceans existed long before most insects. But the vision of crustaceans has a lot in common with that of winged insects. Strange that nature should have endowed creatures of such dissimilar habitat with similar visual equipment.

The best known crustaceans are crab, lobster and shrimp, which dwell in deep-sea water as well as along the continental coasts, and crayfish, which are found in fresh water. Crustaceans can have either simple or compound eyes, and some have both.

The eyes of crustaceans are not the only light-sensitive parts of their bodies. They also have light-sensitive cells called ocelli that occur elsewhere on their bodies. For example, the crayfish has ocelli in its tail. They could be characterized as nature's rearview mirrors. These ocelli can distinguish form and probably movement.

The marine copepod the copelia has a scanning eye, as has already been discussed.

▲

Many crustaceans have their eyes perched on the ends of stalks and can retract them into their carapaces for protection. This arrangement also enables them to see over obstacles.

▶

The eyes of the beautifully marked mantis shrimp from Australia look more like spotlights than eyes.

◀

The unusually marked arrowhead crab carries the pattern of its coloration right into the eyes themselves. With eyes perched on either side of the head, it can see almost completely around itself.

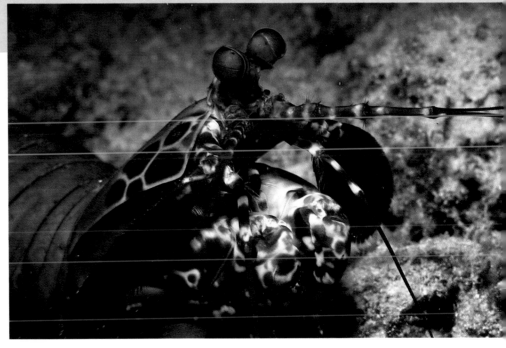

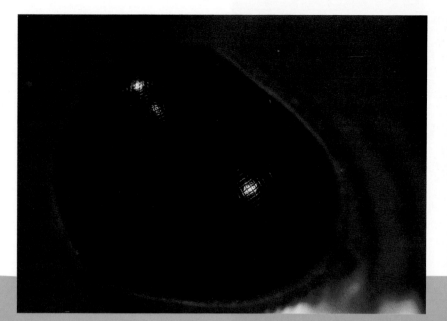

The Compound Eyes of Crustaceans

Crustaceans, like insects, have either apposition or superposition eyes. The apposition eyes are usually found in creatures, like the fiddler crab, that live along the shore, while supposition eyes are more common in those that live in deeper water, like the lobster. The eye of the lobster is the largest compound eye.

However, the vision of many crustaceans differs from that of insects in one very important respect. In the insect compound eye, after light comes through the lens, it is further refracted by the crystalline cone. But many crustaceans have a mirrorlike layer that *reflects* light from all sides of the ommatidia, projecting it onto the retinula cells. This unusual mirrorlike design has been of a special interest to scientists designing modern radio telescopes: Its ability to capture many, many more photons is of particular interest to those studying the night sky.

The ommatidia, which reflect rather than refract light, are much more powerful. While not present in

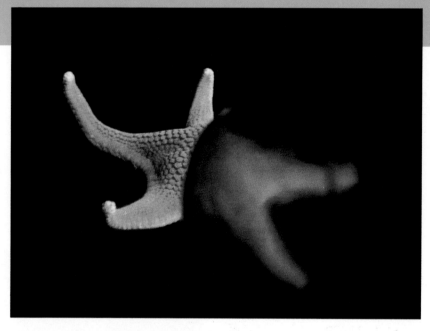

all crustaceans, this visual adaptation is generally found in crustaceans with square-shaped compound lenses, such as lobsters and crayfish.

Nocturnal Crustaceans

The nocturnal crustacean forms its images by superposition—by light from many ommatidia falling on the same retinula cells. This requires less light to form an image but results in an image of lower

quality. No one is very sure of the visual acuity of the lobster.

Again, screening pigment surrounds the sensitive rhabdoms and protects them from excessive glare, moving to expose them in low light and covering them when they are subjected to bright light. There are limits, however, to the protection screening pigment can give. Underwater, the eyes of the Norwegian lobster glow or shine. When it is removed from the water and left on the deck of a ship the glow is lost and the lobster goes blind, because the dark-

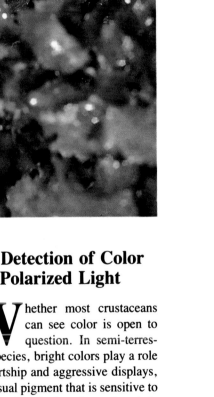

▲

Ghost crabs use their larger claw to send visual signals. They beckon to females and threaten other males.

adapted eye has a limited ability to protect itself from light. All lobsters have similarly dark-adapted eyes, each of which has several thousand large, square-shaped facets.

The visual cells of nocturnal crustaceans are larger than those of their diurnal cousins. But the eyes of the horseshoe crab are unusual in that the rhabdoms actually increase in size at night, becoming several times their daytime size.

Diurnal Crustaceans

Crustaceans who inhabit the shoreline, such as the fiddler crab, have much sharper vision than crustaceans who live in deeper water, due to their apposition compound eyes. They can see stationary objects 20 to 30 meters away and detect a moving figure 100 meters away. Their eyes are on movable stalks, a feature that is quite common in crustaceans and that appeared early in evolution. The stalks allow the eyes to extend upward to see over small obstacles or to retract into the body's carapace for protection.

The Detection of Color and Polarized Light

Whether most crustaceans can see color is open to question. In semi-terrestrial species, bright colors play a role in courtship and aggressive displays, and visual pigment that is sensitive to blues and reds has been found in crayfish. However, they are the only crustaceans thought to be able to perceive color.

It is certain, though, that crabs can detect the plane of polarized light, an obvious aid to navigation. The interior of each rhabdom is made up of

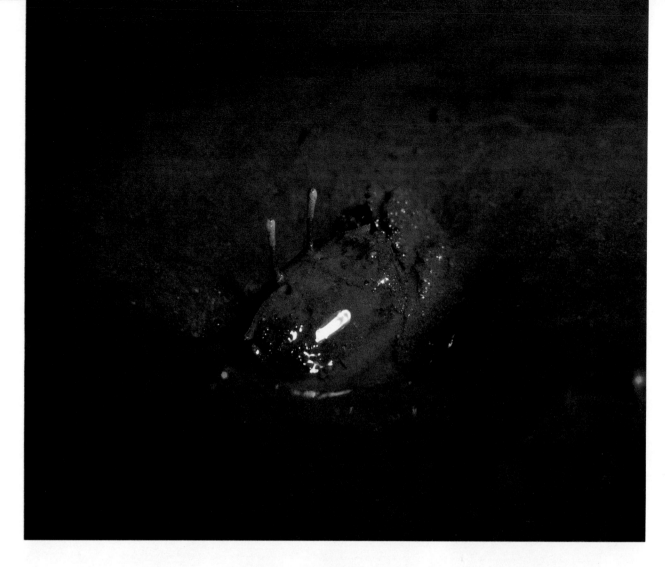

▲

As this Malayan crab emerges from the mud, its eyes, periscope-like, appear first to check the area for predators.

six to eight wedge-shaped rhabdomeres, each of which is composed of tightly packed stacks of microtubules surrounded by visual pigment. These stacks are arranged in parallel layers, but the layers again are structured at right angles. The crustacean is able to detect the path of the light because the photons strike the rhabdomere cells at a specific angle. This ability, of course, is shared with certain insects and cephalopods.

Experiments with horseshoe crabs show that their photoreceptors discharge differently in polarized light than in nonpolarized light, suggesting that this species, too, can detect this type of radiation.

Simple and Compound Eyes

Horseshoe crabs have both simple and compound eyes. The compound are in the sides of the body, while the simple (always more than one) are in the middle area of the shell. Messages from each type of eye are sent to different parts of the brain, the compound eye to the optic nerve and the simple eye to the forebrain; what effect this has on the nature of their function is not known. However, we do know that the simple eye evolved first while the compound eye developed later in evolution. That many crustaceans as well as insects have both types of eyes may be explained by these creatures' early place in the history of evolution. Perhaps nature had not yet decided which eye to pursue.

Unusual Variations

The eyes of some deep-water crustaceans have two distinct sections that actually look in different directions. The upper ommatidia are large, long, nearly parallel facets, while the lower are shorter, smaller units. Since most of the food of deep-sea predators floats down to them from in the richer, sunlit layers of the ocean above, the upper layer is most important.

While the underlying structure of the king crab's eye is similar to that of other crustaceans—i.e., rhabdoms radially arranged below a crystalline cone—in the king crab they lie under a common lens. The optical system is not as much like that of the vertebrate as is the cephalopod's, but it is the only known crustacean to possess a single lens.

6

Cephalopods

Sometimes evolution seems to move in great jumps. The vision of cephalopods may be such an event. Although they are invertebrates, certainly they see as well or better than most animals in the vertebrate world. A cephalopod's head—"cephalo"—extends into a series of feet—"pods"—called tentacles. The members of this family are the octopus, squid, cuttlefish, giant squid and the chambered nautilus.

Perhaps nature has given cephalopods such excellent vision because they are so vulnerable. They have no shells for protection and must rely on visual awareness and speed to escape predation. Cephalopods are a favorite food of many predatory fish and mammals, including man himself. In fact, they make up the bulk of the diet of flesh-eating whales, the Orthodonteci, which may explain why they have not been as successful ecologically as other invertebrate groups: There are only 550 species still in existence, while we have fossilized remains of at least another 9,000.

The Optics of the Cephalopod Eye

The vision of cephalopods is unusual in that it combines a vertebrate-like optical system with invertebrate photoreceptors. Their eyes have an active iris and a rectangular pupil that contracts to a narrow horizontal slit. All other invertebrates have fixed-focus lenses, but cephalopods are able to change the position of the lens relative to the retina

to focus for near and far vision. Contraction of the ciliary muscles around the eyes pulls the lens inward toward the retina for near vision, and raising the internal pressure of the eye pushes the lens outward for far vision. This double focusing system has no parallel in the vertebrate world, and resembles the workings of a camera more than that of our own eyes.

Because the focal length of the lens is so short and the cephalopod's photoreceptors are so long, it can keep objects from a few centimeters away to infinity in sharp focus all the time. For creatures that are always in danger of becoming someone else's dinner, this is a welcome advantage. The lens of the cephalopod is spherical, with a very short focal length (2.5 times the lens radius), which makes for an extremely wide angle of vision. The retina is hemispherical in shape, though longer horizontally than vertically. This particular lens can focus an image at full aperture only if the medium through which the light passes has a refractive index of 1.53 to 1.33—which, fortunately, happens to be that of seawater. (The refractive index measures the ability of a medium to bend light.)

While there are many optical similarities between the advanced vertebrate eye and the eye of the cephalopod, scientists have concluded that one did not evolve from the other. There are so many biological differences that any similarities are thought to be the result of convergent evolution, that is, nature simply applying the same successful solution to two totally independent problems.

Because of its rectangular pupil, many researchers used to think that the cephalopod suffered from horizontal astigmatism. An astigmatism is an imperfection in the corneal surface that causes rays of light from an object to fail to meet in a point on the retina; instead, they spread out into lines, some of which are less distinct than others, causing vision to blur. Astigmatism is widespread in the vertebrate world and is a common human problem. However, unlike any other creature, the cephalopod has two corneal layers, each of which counters the imperfections of the other. In any case, astigmatism is not as grave a problem for underwater creatures, where the cornea plays almost no role in the bending of light rays.

What are we able to tell about the images that appear to the cephalopod eye? Optically they should be excellent, but the screen on which they appear, the retina, causes the cephalopod images to be much coarser than those of human or primate vision. The cephalopod retina contains comparatively few photoreceptors. Remember, the more densely packed the photoreceptors, the greater the acuity of the eye. Think of the human retina as a finer-grain film. Thus, the outlines of objects seen by cephalopods will not be as clear. This may explain the results of experiments with octopi conducted by Stewart Sutherland in 1969, which showed that the animal can recognize only filled shapes rather than outlines. In fact, when they were shown the outline of a previously recognized shape, the octopi were unable to identify it.

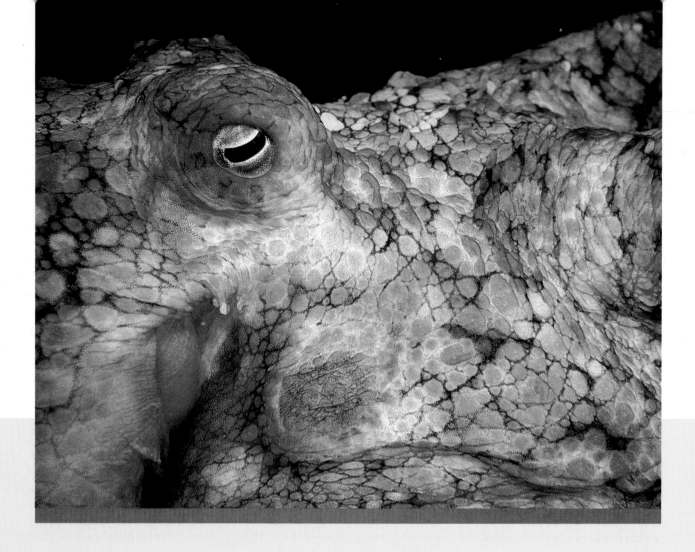

Cephalopod Photoreceptors and Visual Pigment

Cephalopod photoreceptors are large and long, designed to capture as much light as possible, since there is comparatively little light available for vision under water. While the lenses of the cephalopod eye resemble those of the vertebrate eye, their photoreceptors are much like those of other invertebrates. The photoreceptors, called retinula cells, point directly toward the lens in the direction of the incoming light. The outer segment consists of a core and two extended structures called rhabdomeres, each of which contains visual pigment. Generally, there is far less visual pigment in the rhabdomeres of invertebrates than in the rods or cones of vertebrates. Pigment serves another important function in cephalopods: Since they have no lids to protect their eyes, they shield the sensitive photoreceptors from excessive glare by surrounding them with screening pigment. Unlike other invertebrates, they are also able to reduce the amount of light entering the eye by decreasing the size of the pupil.

Cephalopods have two kinds of visual pigment in their retinula cells: One has a maxium wavelength absorption of 475nm, in the blue part of the spectrum, and a second visual pigment with an absorption maximum of 490nm. This second pigment is found deep inside the retinula cells and is more sensitive in dim light than

Octopi and squid are able to change color faster than any other creatures alive.

the 475nm pigment.

The type of visual pigment found in an eye is an important factor in how well the animal sees, particularly underwater, since the ocean acts as a giant filter excluding light of many wavelengths as one goes deeper. For good vision, the wavelength maximum of the animal's visual pigment must closely match the wavelength maxium of the available light, so that creatures that might see well on the surface would be blind at great depths.

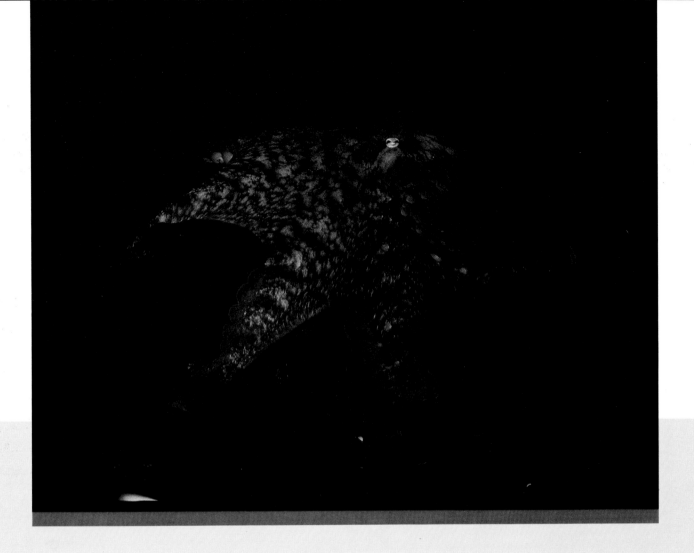

Color Vision In Cephalopods

We know that some color vision can be present where there are two or more visual pigments receptive to different wavelengths of light. The cephalopod does have two such pigments, though one may be contained in a rod and the other in a cone. And it is even possible that color vision in the cephalopod could be discriminated by a combination of rod and cone vision. But the two visual pigments present in the cephalopod's eye are so close that it should indicate that their color vision would be very limited; that is, perception in the blue and blue-green area of the spectrum but little color discrimination in the longer wavelengths.

However, behavioral tests of these creatures have shown that they are able to match their body color to almost any background. In fact, they can change color faster than any other creature alive. The chromatic abilities of most other creatures are subject to hormonal factors and thus are slow, but the cephalopod carries bags of black, yellow and yellow-orange pigment that are controlled by its muscles and can be released almost instantaneously. Additionally, under the black pigment are iridocytes that reflect a greenish light. By mixing these pigments they can match almost any color.

Great care has been taken in the testing of their color vision. Early vision scientists frequently mistook a creature's response to brightness rather than color. Modern testing methods now take this distinction into consideration. Recent experiments have shown that when cephalopods are placed on a gray, white or black background, their color does *not* change, but they do match the background in intensity. What's more, they are able to do this from birth. Yet there are still some modern scientists working in this field who insist that in fact cephalopods cannot see in color, which makes their chromatic abilities even more astonishing. But even if their color vision is of a limited nature, the range of color change remains unexplained. It is rare in vision science for physical and behavioral testing results to be so far apart.

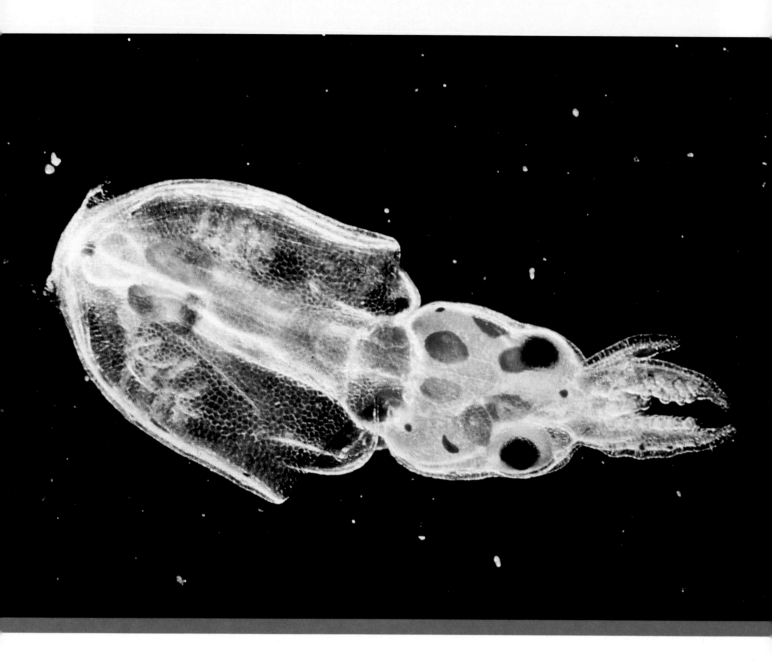

▲

This young loligo squid is only a few days old, but the bags of colored pigment are clearly visible under its skin.

Obviously there are many things that are still unknown.

As with all other invertebrates, the rhodopsin of cephalopods does not immediately fall apart after the absorption of a photon of light, but changes to an intermediate state called metarhodopsin, still capable of absorbing light. Only then does it reabsorb a form of Vitamin A and again become rhodopsin.

The Cephalopod Eye and Polarized Light

It is certain that, like many other invertebrates, cephalopods can detect the plane of polarized light. Rays of light are scattered in traveling through the atmosphere or water, and only those vibrating in one direction can pass. This is called plane-polarization, and it is not visible to the human eye. But the inner walls of the cephalopod's rhabdomeres are covered with perpendicular tubules (to which the visual pigment is attached) that are able to sense the direction in which light is traveling, by detecting the angle at which light strikes them.

Divers sometimes wear polarizing goggles to protect their eyes from the glare of down-welling light. In fact, special lens hoods must be used on underwater cameras or pictures will be flared from above. Certainly the ability of cephalopods to tell the direction in which light is traveling makes them better navigators, but whether the layered tubules also act as an anti-glare device in not yet known.

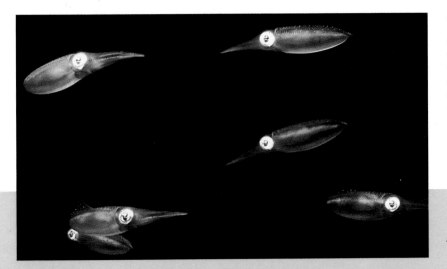

Loligo squid. Bioluminescence is very common in cephalopods, and the larger cephalopods, some of which measure more than 180 feet end to end, have bioluminescent markings around their eyes.

Modern Science and the Octopus

Many scientists have devoted much of their research to the study of cephalopods, in particular the octopus. In fact, much of what we now know about memory comes from a study of the octopus's habits and anatomy.

Shortly after World War II, a group of British scientists led by J. Z. Young started a research station near Naples. They had begun experimenting on cuttlefish in the British Isles, but these creatures did not take well to life in a tank and did not respond well to surgery, so an experimental station studying octopi was established in the warm waters of the Mediterranean. The octopus is not as fine a swimmer as the squid or cuttlefish, preferring to crawl along the ocean floor, but given a tank full of seawater and a few bricks for a home, it tends to settle in.

These remarkable creatures resemble man in that 70 percent of their brains are composed of associative neurons, though they have a mere 300 million brain cells compared to the human brain's many billions. Still, they can be trained to recognize patterns, make choices and learn. Their eyes can scan only vertically and hor-izontally and tend to prefer vertical forms. They appear to be able to measure shapes rather than outlines.

Removal of sections of the octopus brain has shown that there are specific cerebral areas involved in long-term and short-term memory. As a result, we have come to a better understanding of the physiological and chemical reasons that we remember somethings for a few hours and other things for all of our lives.

There was something quite touching in one of the more abstruse scientific tomes I perused while researching this book. When asked how he could tell that the octopus could see at all, a scientist who studies their brains replied, "They stare back at you when you look at them."

Pathways to the Brain

Considering the limited nature of the octopus brain, its ability to recognize forms and to learn is remarkable. Cephalopods generally have a simpler processing system for visual information than do vertebrates. The cephalopod eye is derived from surface ectoderm—skin. The normal layers of nerve cells are missing. There are no layers of bipolar or ganglion cells, which are the vertical links that process information before sending it on to the brain via the optic nerve. Neither are there typical horizontal cells such as glial cells or amacrine cells, but some of these cells *are* found within the brain itself.

The simple brain of the cephalopod has two lobes. The information seen by the left eye crosses completely over to the right brain, and the information from the right eye crosses totally over to the left lobe, at a point known as the chiasma. In more advanced animals, such as primates and man, this crossover is only 50 percent, so that each lobe gets information from both eyes. Vision scientists are puzzled that nature would spend so much effort to come up with a mechanism that seems of so little importance to the daily life of these animals, but it is possible that the arrangement is part of an evolutionary process whose meaning will only become clear in time.

The nerve fibers in cephalopods are much larger than those in humans. In the squid, they are fifty to one hundred times larger, but this does not mean that they are carrying more information than human nerve fibers. Remember that the first computer was enormous, yet its capacities were extremely limited in comparison with the smaller computers of today.

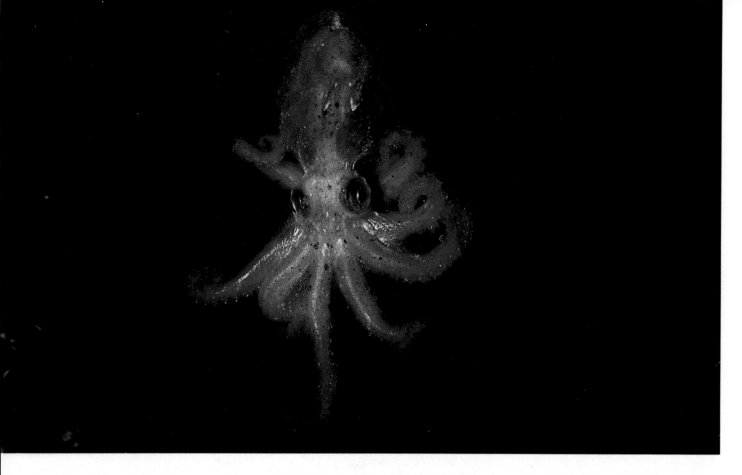

Deep-Water Cephalopods

There are many deep-water squids and octopi of varied and strange appearance. *Vampyroteuthis infernalis*, true to its name, is the strangest of all the cephalopods. With enormous eyes and luminous organs, it lives at depths of 1,000 to 10,000 feet. The body, which has the consistency of a jellyfish, is black and purple. More than half of all cephalopods are bioluminescent, and this includes all deep-water cephalopods.

A great deal of what has been learned about these creatures of the briny deep comes from research conducted and supported by Prince Albert of Monaco, and one is named for his family, the *Grimaldi teuthis*, which is so diaphanous that the lobes of the brain can be seen through its skin. *Bathythannia* has its eyes on stalks, as do many deep-sea teleost fish. Another deep-sea pod found in the South Atlantic, *Sandalops*, has eyes that are pointed obliquely downward, but it

swims with its body slanting upward. Most of these creatures have luminous organs next to or surrounding their eyes. One mid-water squid, *Histioteuthis*, has one eye that points upward and another that points downward; it is evidently watching in both directions at once. The upward eye is five times as large as the downward eye, and its structure is completely different. Again, the eyes are ringed with luminous organs, and some of its discs have claws. Then, of course, there's the largest of them all, *Architeuthis*, the giant squid, which averages 180 feet in length and which, as I mentioned before, has the largest eye in the world. Since it makes its home in equatorial waters and has never been captured by man, all that we know of it comes from studying its remains found in the bellies of whales, the other giants of the ocean. When alive, the giant squid must be a remarkable sight. Jacques Yves Cousteau's navigator reports the sighting of a giant squid during a descent in a mini-sub in the Indian Ocean. Between 160 feet and 500 feet he saw a cloud of plankton. At 800

▲

Half of all cephalopods are bioluminescent, including all those that live in deep water.

feet, he looked through the porthole and saw a huge, unblinking eye staring at him. For some time the two peered at each other, until the giant creature finally swam away.

The Epistulary Body

Cephalopods have a strange additional photoreceptive organ on their backs called the epistulary body. It is yellowish and is extremely large in deep-water pods. Its cells are similar to the photoreceptor cells in the retina that contain rhodopsin. The purpose of this organ is as yet unknown, though it is possible that, like the vestigial third eye of some vertebrates, it is a light clock governing hormonal behavior. For the moment, this is a mystery waiting to be solved.

7 *Fish*

We call our planet Earth, but more than two-thirds of its surface is enveloped by water, and photographs taken from space reveal a shimmering blue globe, the continents appearing only as islands in a gigantic sea.

For this reason alone, it should come as no surprise that, in sheer numbers and types of species, fish dominate the vertebrate world (vertebrates being those creatures who, like ourselves, have an internal skeleton and backbone). Only a fraction of the 302,000,000 cubic miles of oceans, seas, rivers and lakes is habitable. Most fish live on continental shelves and in inland waters. Yet there are strange creatures that manage to survive even thousands of meters below the surface in a world of almost perpetual night, where water is prevented from freezing only by the extraordinary pressure of its own weight.

Fish have managed to survive, and even thrive, in the most turbid water, clouded by decaying vegetation—though one wonders if they can survive man's pollution—as well as in the sparkling waters of the Caribbean. They live and breed in the cold waters of the Arctic and in the balmy Mediterranean, their cold-blooded bodies matching the temperature of the water they inhabit.

For fish, vision is undoubtedly the most important sense, with a few interesting exceptions. They have good perception of form and color. Their eyes are well developed, and the optic lobe, which also controls learned behavior, is the largest part of a fish's brain. While the sense of smell plays a significant role in the search for food—freshwater catfish, eels and sharks have great difficulty

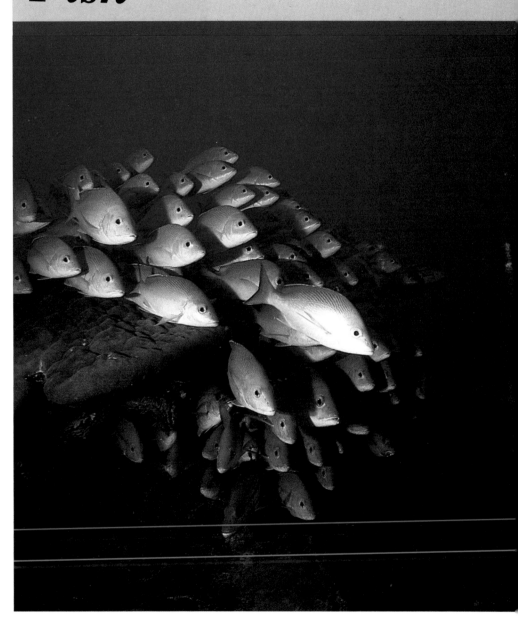

finding food when their nostrils are plugged—most fish are sight-feeders. Vision also plays a major role in the schooling habits of fish, though marine catfish are known to call to one another at night—and if there isn't sufficient light for them to see one another, the school comes apart.

▲
Vision plays an important role in the schooling habits of fish. If the light available for vision goes below a certain level, the school will separate.

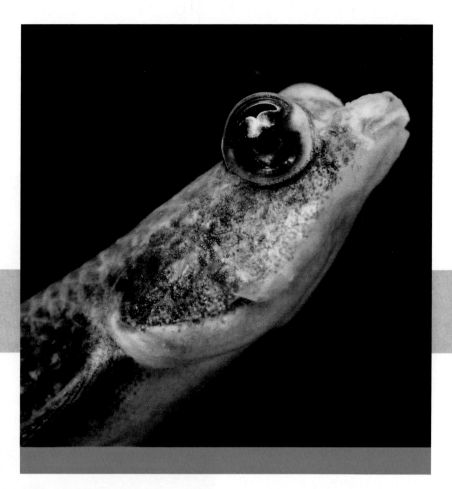

This Caribbean fish, the anableps, is sometimes called the four-eyed fish because of its double retina. It uses the top retina to watch out for enemy seabirds, while with the bottom retina it hunts for fish. Opposite: a photo suggesting how the world might appear to the anableps.

Most fish have a torpedo-shaped body with eyes positioned on either side of the head (members of the flounder family are an exception). This positioning of the eyes is unusual for a predator: Most other predatory animals have their eyes positioned directly in front of their heads. But virtually all fish are prey as well as predators and need a wider angle of vision for their own protection. In contrast, the lion and the leopard have no one to fear but ourselves.

Nature appears to have given vent to its sense of experimentation in the visual mechanisms of fish. Members of the flounder family are born with eyes on either side of their head, but as the larva grow, one side of the skull develops at a faster rate, causing the mouth to become distorted as the eye migrates across the head till both are on the same side. At the same time, the body flattens out. The hammerhead shark has both eyes and nostrils on lobes, or hammers, that extend from either side of the head. The eyes of the larva of the deep-sea fish *Idiacanthus* are perched on the ends of enormously long stalks that contain the optic nerve and eye muscles as well as a cartilaginous rod. And the *Anableps,* a Caribbean fish, has a double retina and double iris, though the upper retina is larger and

its corneal covering is thicker. The top retina watches out for predatory sea birds while the bottom retina searches the water for food.

Vision in Larval Fish

Despite the general excellence of vision in mature fish, that of the offspring is distinctly inferior. This handicap is probably one of the reasons why fish breed in considerable numbers, given the probability that so few will survive.

The transparent bodies of larva cannot shield the nervous system from light, so that, while their powers of image formation are limited, they respond, like plants, to light that strikes their bodies. The eye of the larva and the mature fish of the same species can be vastly different; for example, in the case of salmon, the photoreceptors of the young are structurally different from those of the adult.

Families of Fish

The evolution of fish occupies a space of 400 million years in the history of the earth. The placoderm, an armored fish that dates from Jurassic times, is thought to be the ancestor of all modern fish, including the coelacanth, through which paleontologists trace the descent of man. The coelacanth was long thought to be extinct, but in recent years has been discovered in the waters of South America and the Indian Ocean. Their primitive pituitary glands and hearts are of great interest to scientists.

But it is the teleost, or bony fish, that dominates the waters of the earth, both fresh and salt. Sharks, rays and mantas are all that remain of another group known as the elasmobranchs, who are considered to have left the mainstream of evolution and whose structure is made of cartilage rather than bone. The sturgeon, whose eggs are prized as caviar, is the only survivor of an entire group of fish called chondrosteans; with their large, shiny scales known as ganoids, they are reminiscent of early bony fish. The bowfin, gar and *Amia* are all that remain of the holosteans, again with thick, short scales, probably no different from those of their ancestors who lived millions of years ago.

The *Dipnoi,* or lungfish, have developed primitive lungs that enable them to spend considerable time out of water; an ancient lungfish was probably the ancestor of present-day amphibians. Creatures like the mudskipper fish, which lives in the mangroves of Africa, and the anabas fish of India crawl about on their fins and even court out of the water but must return there to breed. Their vision in air is considerably inferior to their vision in water; once they poke their periscopic eyes above its surface, they become extremely nearsighted.

The lamprey is a very primitive fish, a member of the *Agnatha,* or jawless, fish, that is interesting because it has the vestige of a third eye on top of its head. Called a pineal eye because of its placement near the pineal gland in the brain, this eye is no longer used for vision but serves as a circadian clock influencing hormonal behavior.

Despite some differences in visual mechanisms, the one major factor that influences the vision of all fish is the behavior of light in water. This not only affects the quality of the images they see but also determines the nature of their color vision; for most fish do see in color.

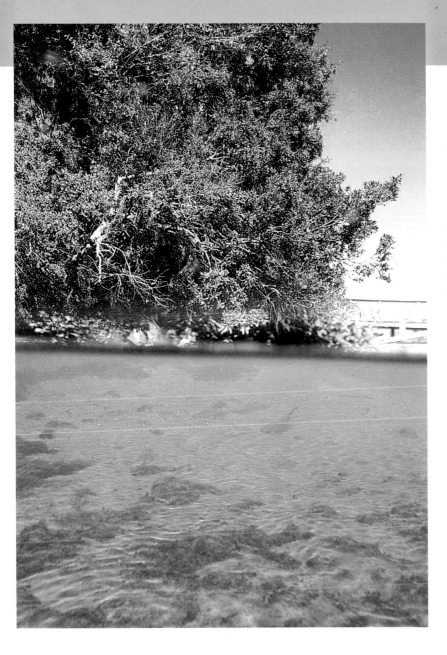

The Spectral Transmission of Light in Water

The most important factor in the vision of all marine life is that even the purest water is a poor transmitter of light. Water acts as a filter; after the first 10 to 15 meters down, all infrared and ultraviolet light is excluded. In addition, all water is filled with tiny particles of decaying vegetable matter and silt as well as plankton, tiny microscopic marine life, all of which absorb certain wavelengths and thus change the water's color. Both the angler and the naturalist have observed that the coloration of salt water differs from that of fresh water. Oceans tend to be blue (like the Mediterranean) or blue-green (like the Baltic). Freshwater lakes and streams, on the other hand, are green or greenish-yellow.

Since only short wavelengths of light can penetrate deep into the ocean, the color vision of saltwater fish is shifted toward the blue end of the spectrum. Freshwater fish that live in shallower streams and lakes are more sensitive to longer wavelengths, the reds. Some of the very shallow freshwater dwellers, such as the perch, have

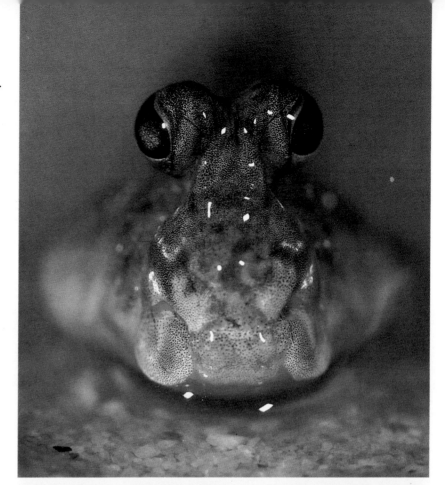

a color sensitivity that peaks around 625nm; this falls into the near infrared, much above what is accessible to the human eye.

As we penetrate more deeply into the oceans, more and more wavelengths of light are filtered out until only those around 475nm remain. This phenomenom is apparent to the human eye underwater: A diver who cuts himself in deep water will find that his blood looks green instead of red. Similarly, fish seen at this depth will appear bluish-gray, though when pulled to the surface they may have red coloring.

Since the background color of seawater is blue or blue-green, yellow, its contrast color, is more visible in the upper levels of the sea. And since freshwater is green or greenish-yellow, reds or oranges are most visible in rivers, lakes and streams. We see corroboration of this fact in the coloration of fish: Yellow tangs and butterfly fish are prominent on tropical reefs, while the red markings on salmon, perch and bass become even more marked during mating seasons.

The Optics of Light in Water

Anyone who swims underwater for any length of time (even though the human eye becomes farsighted without the protection of goggles or a mask) notes the almost-constant glare coming from all directions. Molecules of water scatter individual photons of light, interposing brightness between the sighted object and the eye. The most immediate consequence is that contrast becomes degraded at any real distance, blurring the edges of objects and reducing clarity of vision. However, this is less of a problem for most fish since they are nearsighted anyway; sharks are among the few farsighted exceptions.

The strongest light source in water is above; vision science refers to this as down-welling light. Preda-

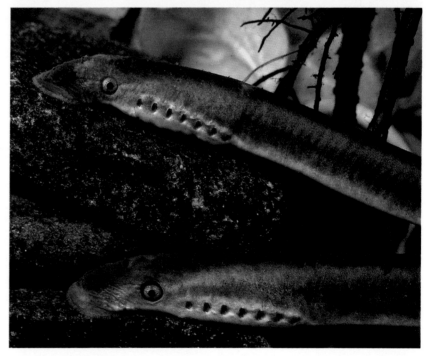

▲
The lamprey is an ancient fish with the vestiges of a third eye on top of its head. Not a true eye, it acts as a hormonal clock, monitoring changes in light levels that affect the body's metabolism.

tory fish look up and see their prey in silhouette; consequently, most fish are countershaded, that is, lighter on the bottom of their bodies than on the top.

Most aquatic light is polarized through contact with the molecules of water and travels vertically in shallow water and horizontally in deep water. Polarized light has the very positive effect of making distant objects more visible and improving fishes' vision. Polarization of light reduces scattering, forcing the light to travel in one direction. Even if fish, unlike many crustaceans and cephalopods, cannot tell from which direction the light is coming, they do benefit from the reduced glare. If it weren't for this polarizing effect, underwater glare would be even more of a problem.

An astute angler is well aware that fish can see above the surface of the water, particularly on a calm day. They have a window on our world of almost 97 degrees, called Snell's window after the Dutch scientist who contributed so much to our knowledge of the nature of light and of refraction in particular. One fish, the archerfish, has mastered the technique of knocking flying insects into the water by spitting at them with great accuracy, notwithstanding the fact that it must compensate for the change in refraction once light enters the water. This is learned behavior and is mastered only through trial and error.

One of the unusual optical properties of water is that objects above the surface appear smaller to fish, while, conversely, objects in the water, when seen from above, look larger. Perhaps this accounts for the extraordinary size of "the fish that got away."

Many fishermen are aware that fish have a window on our world. This window is almost 97 degrees in diameter, named after Snell, the Dutch scientist who contributed so much to our knowledge of the laws of refraction.

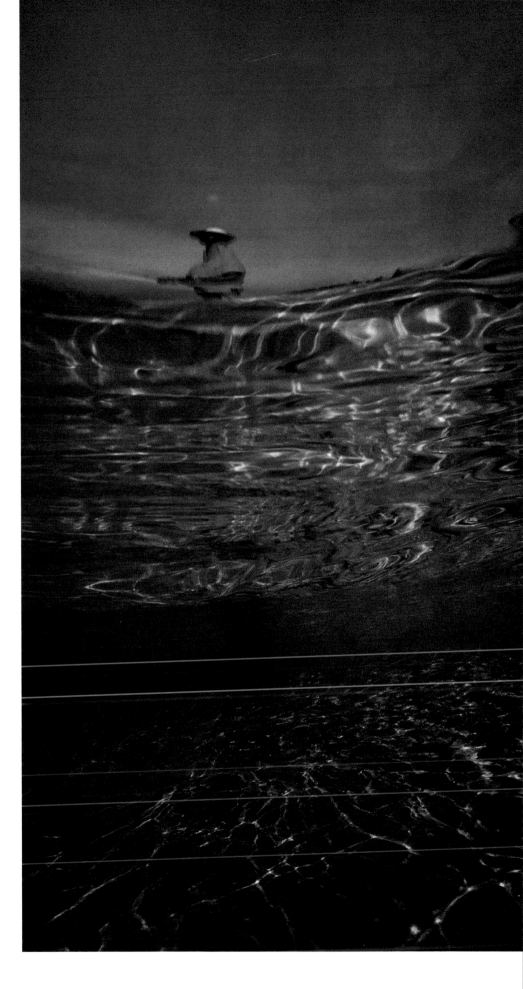

The Eye of The Teleost or Bony Fish

In contrast to all other types of fish, the teleost, or bony, fish is found in both fresh and salt water. Their eye is very similar to the eye of the chondrostean sturgeon and holostean survivors, the gar and *Amia,* and so these others will be included in this section as well; minor variations in their visual mechanism, where they exist, will be mentioned.

All fish have a flattened cornea, in contrast to the curved cornea of land creatures. Certainly a flatter cornea decreases water resistance, but there is another, more important reason for this adaptation: The refractive index of the cornea (the degree to which it can bend light) is almost exactly the same as water's. Thus the cornea of the fish does not have to refract light and is largely protective, keeping out particles of silt or vege-

table matter. The fish also has no need of eyelids as its eyes are constantly bathed in water; our own tears are but a reminder of this experience.

The fish's lens is its most important light-gatherer. Large and spherical, it has a very short focal length (the ratio is 2.55 times the radius of the lens). Perhaps to compensate for the lack of assistance from the cornea, the fish lens has the highest refractive index of any vertebrate lens. However, its extreme round shape is the cause of the fish's nearsightedness. The eye is able to accommodate somewhat for far vision by pushing the lens away from the retina; for near vision, the lens is pulled closer. This accommodative mechanism resembles the mechanics of a camera more than does the human eye.

The bony fish glides through the water wide-eyed no matter how much light is present, its iris and pupil for-

ever fixed in an open position. Fish kept in darkened tanks and suddenly exposed to light fall to the bottom stunned and blinded; they are unable to move for a considerable length of time. The absence of what is called a pupillary response, such as our own, where the iris opens and closes very swiftly in response to changes in light intensity, makes fish extremely vulnerable to what is called dazzlement. Remember, the eye is the only direct opening to the central nervous system for any animal.

How does nature protect the fish eye from glare? With a very slow

Through trial and error, the archerfish learns to capture insects that fly slightly above the water by squirting them and knocking them down. This is more complex than it appears. Because of the refraction of light in water, the insect is not where it appears to be to the fish's eyes.

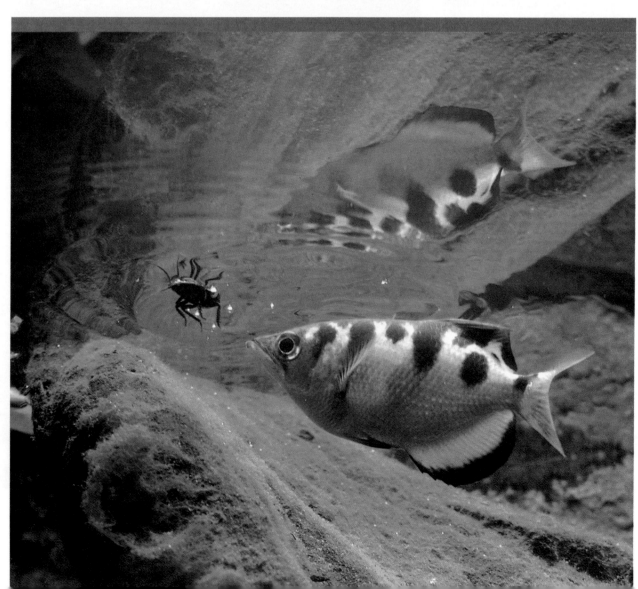

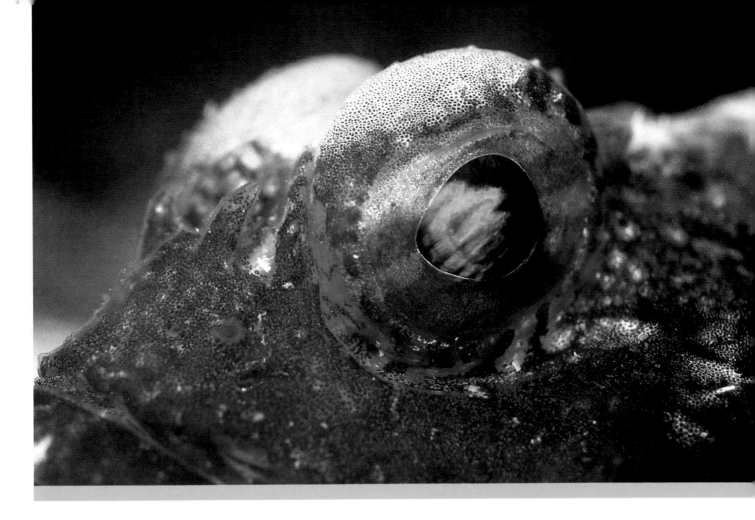

▲

Iridescent corneas are found in insects as well as fish, neither of which can close their eyes. Only certain wavelengths of light can pass through, and others are strongly reflected in wildly glittering colors. The seemingly transparent cornea acts as a sunshade.

process of "retinomotor responses" that takes place over a period of several hours and limits the movement of fish in a vertical column of water until its eyes go through a light or dark adaptive process.

The light-adaptive part of the process involves the movement of screening pigment, which surrounds the sensitive photoreceptors and shields them from the light. At the same time, the photoreceptors themselves, rods and cones, shrink in size. During dark adaptation, the screening pigment draws back and the photoreceptors expand. The fish's eye apparently has a memory for the sunlight changes that take place in water. Researchers who have varied the tim-

ing of light changes in tank experiments have noted that the fish begin to adapt based on previous experience.

This may be one reason why fish frequently remain in a specific layer of water or only rise to feed at twilight. Researchers have remarked that fish that feed on plankton have excellent vision and feed during the day. Predatory fish feed during twilight, and their eyes tend to have poorer pattern formation as well as less color vision.

Bottom fish and those that live in shallow waters have more complex corneas that are divided into two parts, the cornea itself and what is called a spectacle. The spectacle is an additional clear covering that overlays the cornea, protecting the eye from silt and other abrasive materials. Fish with spectacles frequently also have yellow filters in their lenses to filter out the shorter wavelengths. (These are fish that live in shallow water.) This is only one of the reasons why we

consider the bony fish to be the most advanced of all fish; the more ancient sturgeon still has oil droplets in its individual photoreceptors, nature's first light-filtration system.

Iridescent corneas are common to many diurnal bony fish, particularly bottom and shallow-reef fish, though they are found even in pelagic fish, those that dwell at extremely deep levels of the ocean. They are particularly common in fish that also have yellow filters. For some time it was thought that these acted as a polarizing filter, but modern theory regards them as a sophisticated sunshade to minimize the glare from down-welling light. Iridescence results when light passes between two transparent materials with varying refractive indexes. Some wavelengths of light are strongly reinforced, giving rise to a wildly glittering rainbow of color, while others are canceled out. The iridescent cornea takes advantage of this cancellation effect, preventing wavelengths of light that cause excessive

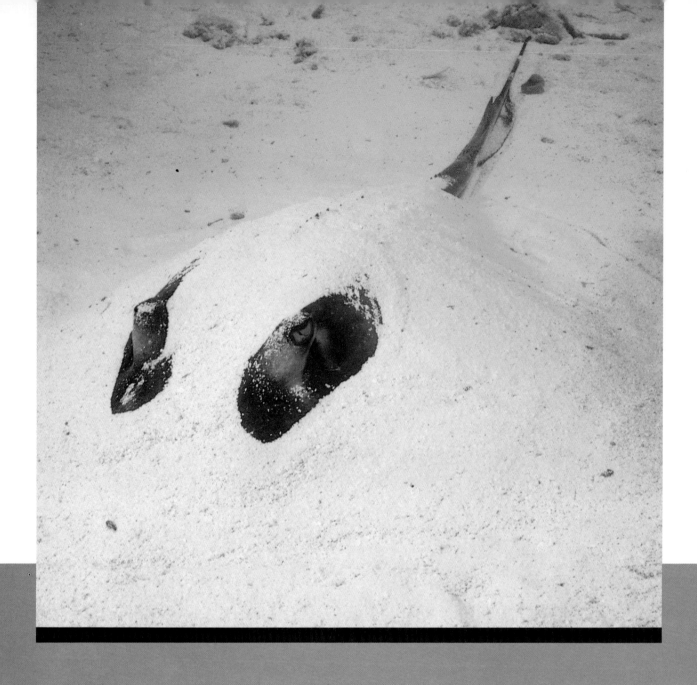

▲ ▲

Rays and flounder are the only fish to have both eyes on one side of their heads. Both also have a filigree-like pupillary flap that extends over the eye and protects it from the glare of down-welling light.

glare from entering the eye but allowing enough light to pass for image formation.

The silvery coloration of many fish is created by their iridescent scales. Each scale reflects one-third of the spectrum; where three scales overlap, all colors are canceled out, leaving a mirrorlike effect. This effect forms an important part of protective coloration in fish, since their bodies then reflect the background in which they swim, breaking up the outline of their bodies and making them more difficult for predators to see.

The tapeta of fish are superior to those of land animals. Made of guanine, the same substance that forms the basis of the fish's shiny scales, the cells of the tapeta of bony fish are found in the retina, except in sharks and sturgeons, where the tapeta are buried in the choroid layer behind the retina. Such choroidal tapeta have specular reflectors with a layer of thin, parallel crystals. In the sturgeon, the crystals are hexagonal, thick at the center and thinner toward the periphery of the eye. Specular reflectors give off sharp rays of reflected light. In contrast, the tapeta of most bony fish are small spheres and the light they reflect is more diffused.

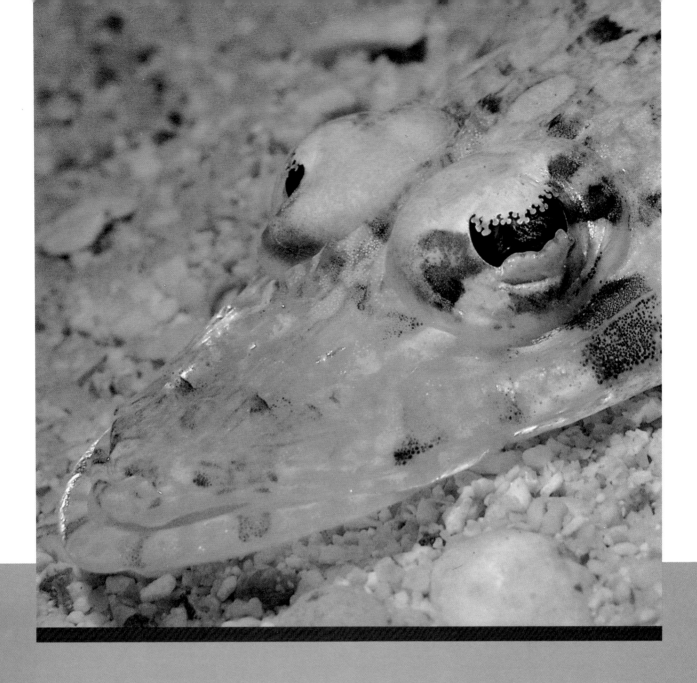

The organization of tapetal cells also varies. Non-grouped cells, common to most deep-sea fish, are found scattered in a single layer in front of the tapetum so that light is reflected only once before it is absorbed or lost. In the more-evolved teleost fish, the photoreceptor cells are formed into distinct groups separated from one another by layers of reflecting tapetal cells. Thus photons may be reflected many times, more than doubling the photoreceptors' chances of capturing them.

Bottom-Dwelling Bony Fish

The most unusual are the members of the flounder family (e.g., sole, halibut, turbot), with their flattened bodies and migrating eye. (In the case of one member, *Psettodes,* the eye does not quite make it to the top of the head.) These are the only predatory bony fish to have eyes on one side of the head. In some cases, they stick up peri-scope-fashion. They are the only fish to have any extensive binocular vision.

Glare from down-welling light is obviously such a problem for some fish, given the slow pace of the retinomotor responses, that bottom fish have an additional visual mechanism to protect them from glare; this is the operculum, a filagree-like pupillary body that extends over the top of the eye. They share this type of light guard with the ray, which also has its eyes on top of the head.

Tropical Marine Fish

Most tropical reef fish live in the upper regions of the water; at this depth, colors are more like those seen in the air. The fish themselves are a riot of bright colors. These fish are extremely territorial and aggressive; color provides important signals. The wild and glorious colors of the harlequin, the green-spotted boxfish and the clown fish advertise their presence, warning off intruders and attracting mates. Parrot fish distinguish males from females through their coloring, and when an insufficient number of males are available, females change both their sex and their color.

Pattern recognition may be more important to reef fish than to any others. Various butterfly fish all have the same basic body design, but their patterns differ from one another in minute details: small patches of dots, zigzags, stripes and patches. The male and female of one family must be able to recognize each other from such small variations in markings if they are to make a fertile union. Remember that pattern recognition may be the first step in abstract thinking.

Changes in Color

Some fish can camouflage themselves by changing color to match their background. The Nassau grouper has at least eight different motile patterns. Such a highly complex defensive mechanism could not have evolved but for the visual abilities of predators.

Fish change color via signals from the central nervous system, a system very much like the advanced chromatophores of the cephalopods, though the latter can do it faster. The change is activated neurally, signal-

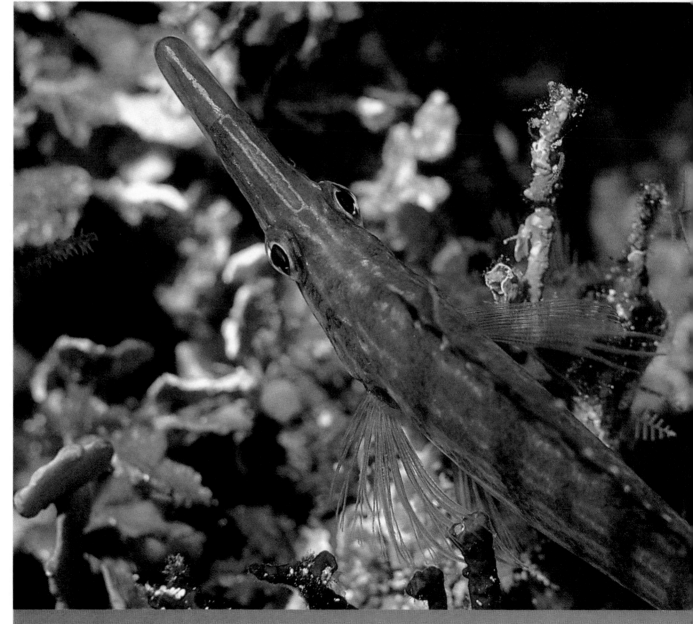

ing the muscles to expand bags of pigments contained within the skin; a system, by the way, that is much more rapid than the hormonal signals sent via the bloodstream in some insects and amphibians.

Some color changes last for only a moment. The leaping marlin is suddenly colored by brilliant silver and gold bands. When the amberjack becomes excited, the stripe that runs through its eye darkens; the freshwater perch goes pale when frightened. Color change is either a signal or a disguise, but in either case it is a tribute to the excellence of fishes' color vision.

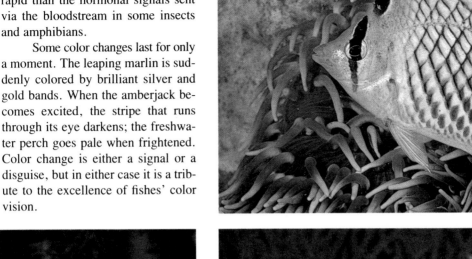

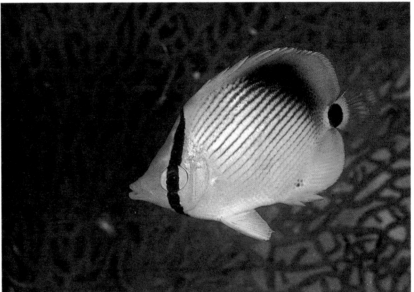

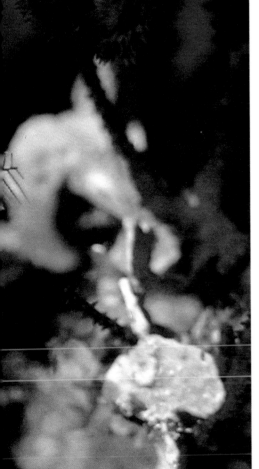

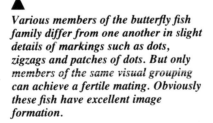

▲
Various members of the butterfly fish family differ from one another in slight details of markings such as dots, zigzags and patches of dots. But only members of the same visual grouping can achieve a fertile mating. Obviously these fish have excellent image formation.

◄
The eyes of the longnose hawkfish are located so far back on either side of the head that they afford an extremely wide angle of vision but little frontal binocularity.

Freshwater Bony Fish

Most freshwater fish are sight-feeders, so turbidity is a more serious problem for them than for saltwater fish. Extremes of decaying vegetation and pollution cause the cornea to cloud and ultimately blind the fish.

Pike, whose eyes are positioned on either side of their head, are endowed by nature with sighting grooves that extend from their eyes to the tip of their snout, improving their binocular vision. The brown trout is unusual in that it is thought to be able to focus on a near and a far object at the same time. It has an egg-shaped

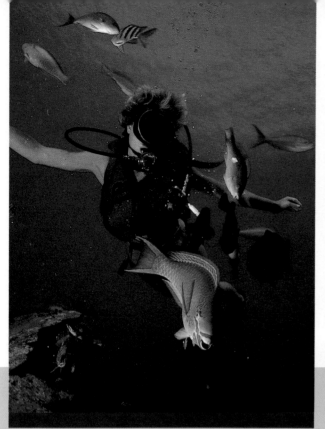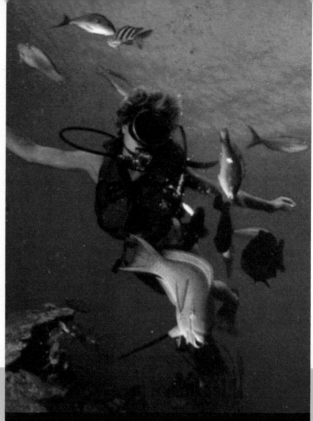

▲

Image formation in sharks is more limited than our own. First, they have few retinal cones and most have no color vision. Second, their rod receptors are larger and fewer in number than ours, so that the picture they have of the world is much coarser than our own. Here we see a diver as she would appear to another human, and how she might appear to a shark.

lens that points directly at the retina, so that separate parts of an image are read in different areas of the retina. Its vision is best in the area at right angles to its eyes, and it probably has a large blind spot dead ahead. There is even the possibility that it may suffer from split vision. The fish compensates for this problem by turning its head from side to side as its swims to get a better look at what is in front of it. In general, trout are excellent sight-feeders, attacking their prey head on and swallowing them head first. Bass also have excellent vision and even superior color discrimination, though size may be a more important factor in their predation than is color.

Vision of Sharks, Rays, and Mantas (The Elasmobranchs)

Sharks, rays and mantas have the same ancestor as other fish, the placoderm, but their eyes have distinct variations. For example, the eyes are extremely small in relation to body size (though certainly not as proportionately small as the eyes of whales, which are not fish but deep-sea mammals). Also, sharks, rays and mantas are farsighted. Their lenses are so perfectly graded that they suffer from very little astigmatism. This is not to say that their vision is superior to that of other fish. It is probably inferior, for they have fewer photoreceptors and hardly any cone photoreceptors, and most see only in black and white. As with most nocturnal creatures, their eyes have sacrificed acuity for light sensitivity. Theirs is a grainy and indistinct picture of the world, though they do see form at a distance more clearly than do bony fish.

Like ourselves, elasmobranchs have what is called the pupillary response, meaning that the iris is mobile, opening and closing depending on the amount of available light, but this process occurs far more slowly than our own. Scientific historians believe that the pupillary response was transmitted to amphibians—and after a long road to ourselves—not through the elasmobranchs but via an ancient fish that no longer exists, the crossopterygian.

Since the elasmobranch pupillary response is much slower than our own, some of them have additional aids to prevent dazzlement. Sharks that hunt in daylight, as well as rays and mantas, have an operculum (a filagree-like protective flap over the pupil) that they share with members of the flounder family. Some deep-sea elasmobranchs, such as rays and the blue shark, also have nictitating membranes, opaque eyelids, also found in some birds, that decrease the amount of light entering the eye without completely obscuring vision. In addition, deep-sea sharks are able to mask the reflecting crystals of their tapetum when there is too much light.

It is only recently that scientists have come to believe that some sharks can detect color; the lemon shark is one such creature. Since the pale, still eyes of sharks detect so little color, this may be one reason why their body coloration is so bland, lacking the vivid markings of other fish. Most sharks have what is called rod-rich vision, that is, almost all rod. Cones, where they exist in sharks, improve contrast detection but add nothing to color discrimination. The photoreceptors of some deep-sea sharks are

▼

The eyes and nostrils of the hammerhead shark are located at the ends of two long lobes on either side of the head, giving these fish a rather strange appearance. These fish have a large blind spot dead ahead.

so primitive, in addition, that it is impossible to distinguish rod from cone.

As creatures move to deeper levels of the sea, nature makes the eye larger and larger in an effort to capture the available light, but suddenly a "quit point" is reached and members of the same species that live at lower levels suddenly have much smaller eyes and become more dependent on other senses. *Etmopterus,* a mid-ocean shark, has extremely large eyes, but in *Laemargus,* a chimaera shark of the abyss, the eyes have become considerably smaller.

Like all other animals, sharks must ingest carotenoids to make Vitamin A_1. Since sharks are predators, this cannot come from plants but must come from other creatures. For some reasons the livers of some sharks contain an abnormally high amount of Vitamin A; until recently, in fact, hammerhead sharks were fished commercially for this very reason.

Deep-Sea Fish

The first descent in a bathysphere was made off the coast of Bermuda by a man named Lucas Beebe, who described the change in coloration of the water as his vessel went deeper and deeper. There came a moment when the water changed from blue to dark gray and then another where everything went black. For a while it remained dark, and then it was, he said, as if the stars came out. He was seeing the phenomenom we call bioluminescence, the ability of some animals to create their own light.

It is a far different light than that which we make with light bulb or flame; it is cold light. Ninety percent of the energy used goes to create the light itself, while only 10 percent becomes heat. The molecular activity of a light bulb or candle produces almost exactly the reverse.

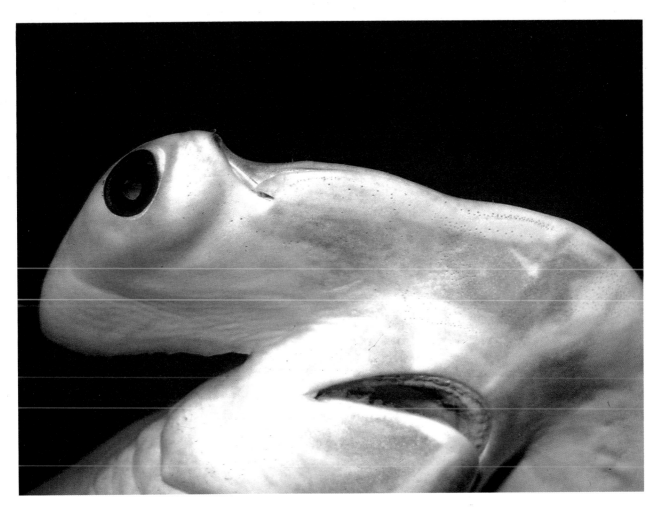

Were it not for bioluminescence, it is probable that most deep-sea fish would be blind. (There are blind fish, such as the *Pygidiid* catfish and the *Amblyopsid,* but they live in caves and are not deep-sea fish; their larva are born with eyes but lose them as they mature.) Certainly the abyss is populated with some of the strangest-looking creatures known to man: the gulper eel, the ceratoid angler fish and chimaera sharks are truly bizarre. But the strangest of all vertebrate eyes belongs to a deep-sea fish called ipnops.

As with most deep-sea fish, the eyes of ipnops are found on top of the head. No plants grow at these levels, so all the inhabitants are carnivorous, frequently scavengers of what floats down from above. The head is flat under transparent roof bones; below it the organs have become platelike. All traces of a lens have vanished; the eye is simply a flattened fibrous tunic and a retina. Each eye has 250,000 rods connected by an optic nerve to the brain. Obviously, this creature has no image-forming powers.

Ipnops represents an extreme. But the shape of the eyes of most deep-sea fish have undergone an important change; they have become tubular, a configuration they share with a far different creature but one who also must capture as much light as possible, the nocturnal owl. In both cases, the eyes have become tubular because there is no space left in the head for them to expand in a circular form. By changing the shape of its eye, the ipnops keeps the relationship between lens and retina at the ratio of 2.55 times the radius of the lens, the same as all other fish. But unlike the owl, deep-sea fish have developed an additional retina; the main retina is responsible for near vision, while the smaller accessory retina to the side of it is used for far.

Cones are rare in deep-sea fish, though there is one known exception with almost pure cone vision, osmosudis. Deep-sea teleosts are thought to use their cones for communication with other members of their species, as they would be particularly sensitive to bioluminescent light given off by members of their own kind.

The rods of deep-sea fish are long and slender and are found in very large numbers, from 100,000 to several million per square inch. They have

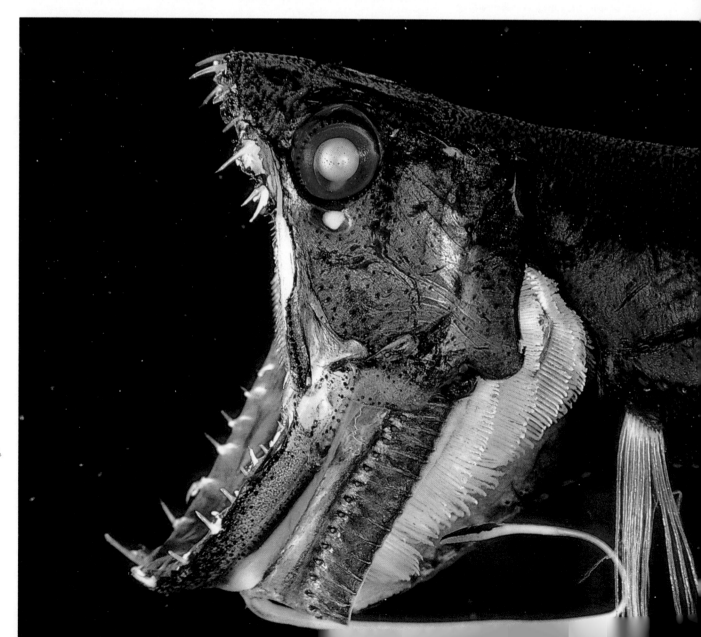

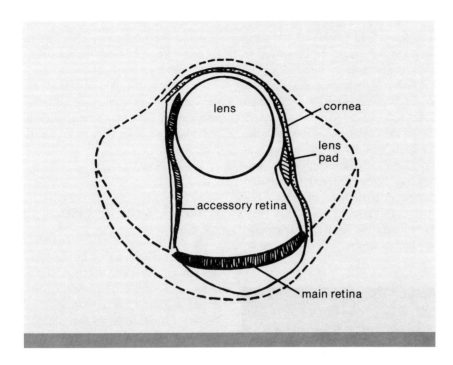

The eyes of deep-sea fish, like those of nocturnal birds, have become tubular in an effort to capture more light. However, the deep-sea fish has an additional retina that it uses for peripheral vision, something that is not found in the nocturnal bird.

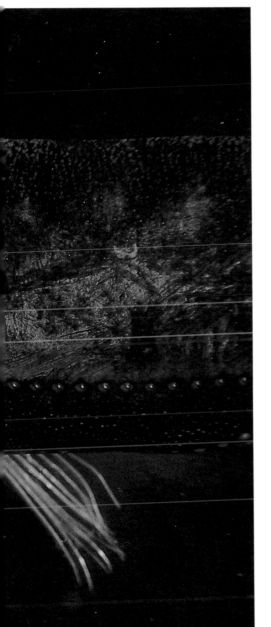

This deep-sea hatchetfish lives in the abyssal region of the ocean where there is little light. Its eyes have slowly migrated to the top of its head, although when the fish is first hatched, they appear at the sides of the head.

the most highly sensitive retinas of any creature alive, but if any image is to be formed, the fish needs a large pupil as well. Large deep-sea fish that have both big eyes and numerous photoreceptors are found at between 200 and one thousand meters. Any deeper, the fish become very small.

Despite its chilling appearance, a deep-sea hatchetfish is only three to four inches in size. Because of the intense water pressure, their skeletons are very light and can be seen through their almost-transparent bodies. They have weak jaws but very sharp teeth. When hatched, their larvae have their eyes facing forward, but as they mature, the eyes move to the top of the head.

Certainly finding a mate in these dark conditions is difficult. In one deep-sea anglerfish, *Protocornus*, the female carries her considerably smaller mate along with her, attached to her body. Some carry more than one.

Chryopsin, a golden visual pigment, is found in the photoreceptors of deep-sea fish. It is sensitive, as one might expect, only to wavelengths in the blue end of the spectrum; these are the only wavelengths that can penetrate to that level.

The most common colors of bioluminescent light are white, blue and blue-green. Rarely are they red or red and green; two deep-sea fish, pachystomias and aristomias, are rare exceptions and have some red-sensitive photoreceptors; the few deep-sea crustaceans that emit red light form part of their diet.

Bioluminescent light is created from an enzyme, luciferase, which is activated by exposure to oxygen. Luciferase is produced by photic cells, luminous excretions or bacteria. Bioluminescence is not only a deep-sea phenomenon, however; the flashlight fish of the Red Sea carries symbiotic bioluminescent bacteria in grooves beneath its eyes and uses them as a light to find food as it feeds at night. There are also bioluminescent algae, fungi and insects, but the phenomenon is most prevalent among deep-sea creatures, who dwell in constant darkness.

Most deep-sea bioluminescent light is produced by bacteria that exist only in salt water, but scientists have been unable to figure out how the bacteria are passed from adult to larval fish. In the adult, the bacteria are carried in the gut or pore, which the fish can open or shut at will. Some fish and squid that emit their own bioluminescent excretions are said to be able to match the same wavelength as down-welling light. Consider the magnitude of what is involved in this: The photon of bioluminescent light that is emitted must vibrate with exactly the same frequency as the photon that descends through the water, a frequency measured in *billionths* of a meter; light created by our own sun or a distant star is matched by a living piece of protoplasm, an inorganic, random process replicated by creatures with very little brain power. It makes one think.

In a way, the patterns of bioluminescent light given off by some deep-sea fish might be compared to colored markings in other fish. The rod vision of these creatures responds to the background light while their cones react to the higher wavelength bioluminescence. Some fish even use the glow emitted by the bacteria as bait: One deep-sea angler fish suspends a barbel covered with bioluminescent bacteria in front it. When another fish goes for the bait, it finds itself inside the angler fish's mouth. Similarly, the deep-sea scaly dragon-

fish seeks its prey with a long lure of skin that hangs from its chin and is coated with symbiotic bacteria that glow with a yellow light.

Light in the abyssal regions of the sea serves as another startling example of nature's infinite ingenuity in providing creatures with an image of their world.

Color Vision in Fish

A fish's color vision is influenced primarily by the type of water and depth at which it lives. As has already been mentioned, saltwater fish have their color vision shifted toward the shorter wavelengths, while freshwater fish have theirs shifted toward the longer-wavelength light.

Color vision in any creature occurs because nature is trying to improve the animal's ability to detect contrast. The first type of visual pigment found in its photoreceptors generally matches the overall back-

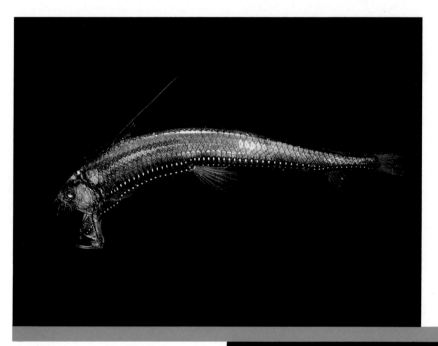

▲ ▶
Fish of the abyssal region of the sea frequently give off signals that are visible only to members of their own species. Others use bioluminescent lures as bait to catch prey. Here we see Sloane's viperfish shown in normal state and giving off its luminous display. This fish lives at depths of 1,500 to 9,000 feet, but migrates vertically twice a day and can be found near the surface during the night.

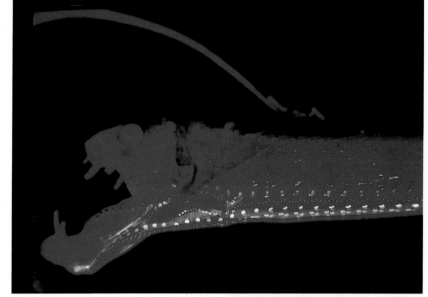

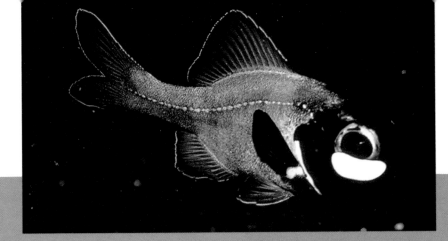

◀

This flashlight fish is a nocturnal feeder and uses the bacteria it carries in its eyes as a lamp. The bacteria in turn live off the fish's blood supply.

The vision of many freshwater fish is shifted so far toward the longer wavelengths that some of them can see in the infrared area of the spectrum. Here is an underwater scene shot with infrared film, which gives us some idea of what the color shift might be like.

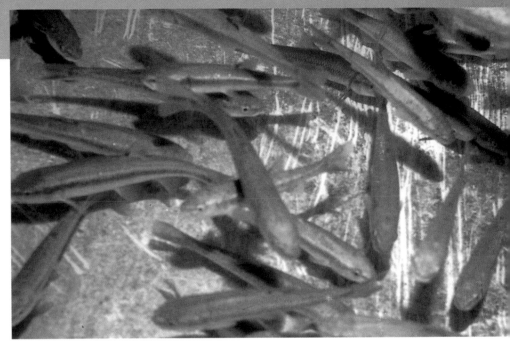

ground light of its environment. This enables the animal to see a dark object against the background. But in order for it to see a light object, another visual pigment must also be present.

As you can see from the adjacent illustration, the peak wavelength absorbencies are represented by curves rather than sharp points, so that when we speak of an animal having a visual pigment with a wavelength maximum of 500nm, that does not mean that its visual pigment absorbs *only* photons that vibrate at a frequency of 500nm; it is also absorbing photons that are slightly under and slightly above. (See "Color Vision in Mammals" in Chapter 11.)

When a second visual pigment is added, you will also note from the illustration, the two have an area of overlap. This overlap is of major importance to color vision because it is in the area of overlap that the creature is best able to discriminate differences in wavelength, i.e., differences in color. Color vision vastly improves the ability of an animal to separate an object from its background. In the case of fish this is particularly important. Unlike land animals that can separate an object from its background by the difference in brightness, fish must contend with the optical properties of water that have already been mentioned; molecules of water scatter photons of light, producing ambient brightness (vision science calls it veiling light) between the eye and an object. Since fish cannot rely on differences in brightness, they are even more dependent on color vision than are land animals.

Most fish have some sort of color vision. Generally they are dichromats, that is, they have two types of visual pigment in their photoreceptors. Creatures with more advanced color vision have three types of visual pigment; this expands considerably the range of colors that they can see. There are trichromatic fish. The goldfish is one, a member of the carp family called *Cyprinidae* which also includes a wilder member called the rudd. But of the goldfish's three color receptors, the red-sensitive cone is dominant. This is not typical of other animals. Since all cones share the same synaptic pathway with the other color cells, the red-sensitive cells can mask or inhibit the other color messages and the vision of these fish shifts toward the red end of the spectrum so that objects that look yellow

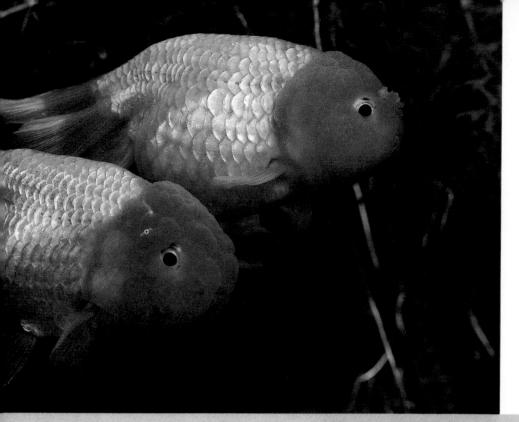

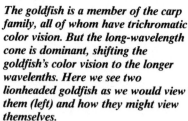

The goldfish is a member of the carp family, all of whom have trichromatic color vision. But the long-wavelength cone is dominant, shifting the goldfish's color vision to the longer wavelenths. Here we see two lionheaded goldfish as we would view them (left) and how they might view themselves.

to us appear orange to them. However, since members of this group frequently live in turbid water, they often suffer from clouded corneas which impinge on the quality of their color vision.

Some fish have more color receptors in one part of the eye than another. The guppy has its color photoreceptors concentrated on the top of its eye; during mating, the male positions itself slightly above the female so that its color markings are more visible to her.

The presence of cones in a fish's retina does not mean that it has color vision; there may be too few. Also, some fish have what are called double cones in their retinas, but it is generally believed that these photoreceptors act as a light-gathering tool rather than imparting some sort of special color ability.

While the visual pigment chryopsin predominates in deep-sea fish, other types of visual pigment are found in freshwater and other saltwater fish. Rhodopsin is the visual pigment of the rods in saltwater fish and porphyropsin that of freshwater fish. As might be expected, porphyropsin

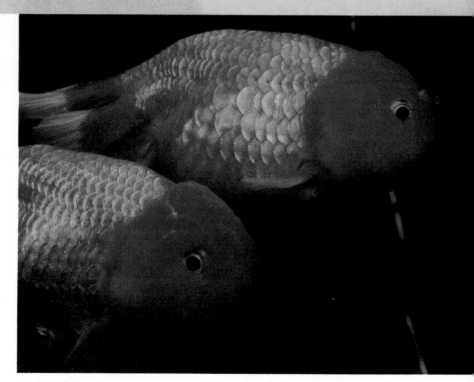

is more sensitive to longer wavelengths (the red end) of the spectrum. Each pigment has its own particular coloration. Chryopsin is golden, while rhodopsin appears reddish when associated with rods and violent when in cones. Porphyropsin on the other hand is a deep purple.

Navigation in Fish

Despite their inability to perceive polarized light, fish are formidable navigators; they sometimes move thousands of miles through the sea. Of particular note is the migration of two different fish, each of which makes a significant change in habitat for a considerably long period and then a return to the original habitat where it spawns and dies. While we are not sure that visual cues are involved in the migration itself, it is thought that the migration is inspired by a change in light intensity when the fish reaches a specific level of maturity. Significant changes also occur in the visual mechanism of the eye.

Salmon are born in streams and slowly make their way to the ocean, where they may live from two to five years before returning to the same stream to spawn and die. In alevins—tiny salmon—porphyropsin is the dominant visual pigment, but the proportion of porphyropsin to rhodopsin reverses as they make their way to the sea.

The process occurs in eels in reverse. After hatching in salt water off the Caribbean island of Anguilla (the Spanish name for eel), the tiny glasslings make their way to the rivers and streams of Europe and America, where they live for about seven years before returning to the Caribbean to spawn and die. In the eel, the visual pigment is first a form of rhodopsin, then changes to porphyropsin while the animal lives in fresh water, then becomes deep-sea rhodopsin as the eels return to the Caribbean.

The change in the structure of the eye of the eel during periods of metamorphosis is even more dramatic than that of the salmon. During its life in freshwater, the eyes are very small. Before scientists realized that the river eel was not a mature creature, they were astounded at the number of rods packed into such a small space. But upon maturity, which occurs at about seven years of age, the eel's skin becomes a silvery color and its eyes become extremely large for its body. The smaller eyes, nearsighted in the vegetation-filled streams and rivers, become farsighted in the sea. In fresh water, the eel has not required great clarity of vision, but with its much larger eyes, it is now ready for the journey through the ocean.

▼

The male sockeye salmon becomes even redder during the mating season. Red is the color most visible in fresh water, while yellow is most visible in salt water.

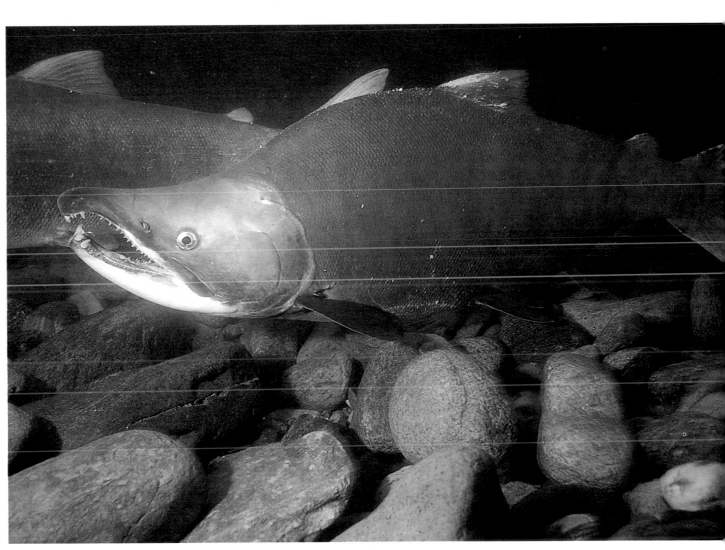

8

Amphibians

The earliest amphibians who poked their heads out of a pond and tried to make their way to a larger pond did not see well at all. Breathing through new lungs and supporting themselves on fins, they looked at the world through the flattened corneas of fish. The new terrestrial environment could only have been one great nearsighted blur.

Perhaps the first amphibians resembled a fish that still exists and still exhibits these same traits: the mudskipper of Africa. Walking on its fins, the mudskipper can even climb into the limbs of mango trees that overhang ponds—imagine a tree full of fish! It spends hours out of water, even courts out of water, but must return there to breed.

The name *amphibian* means "double life." Though conceived and hatched in water, these creatures spend their adult lives on land, with a few purely aquatic exceptions. Survival on land meant that nature not only had to develop a new breathing device, lungs, but also to make a major change in the structure of the eye, if the first land dwellers were to be able to see farther than the tips of their noses.

Let us quickly recap the difference in the way light behaves in water and in air. Light travels in a straight line unless it encounters a more dense medium. As it penetrates the new medium, it can be slowed, which causes a change in direction; it bends if it hits the surface at an angle. The scientific term for this bending is *refraction*. A photon wending its way to earth from our sun or a distant star meets very little opposition till it reaches the earth's atmosphere, where droplets of dust and moisture scatter some of the photons. Nonetheless, many photons continue on unimpeded.

A photon penetrating water is suddenly surrounded by large molecules through which it must pass. As a result, a great deal of energy is lost and the photon changes direction, or refracts, markedly. We say the refractive index of water is high, meaning that it refracts light greatly.

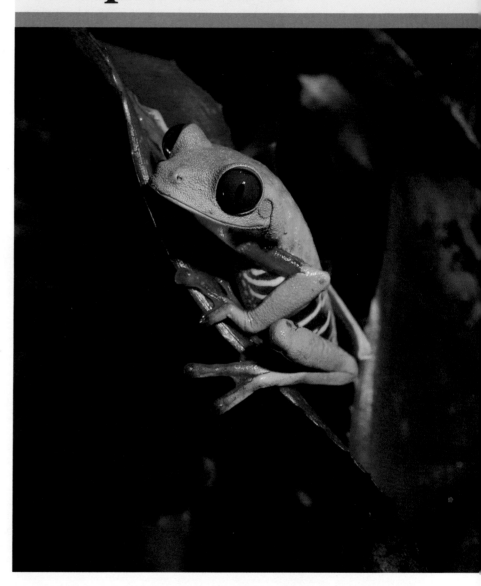

▲

Like other frogs, the red-eyed tree frog of Costa Rica has eyes that protrude from the top of its head, giving it a very wide angle of vision.

Nature took advantage of the refractive quality of light and created an organ, the eye, that could use its own physical structure also to bend light. First the cornea and then the lens force photons to strike the retina, where individual photoreceptors absorb them and convert them into the images that the eye sees. The first part of the eye encountered by a photon is the clear tissue we call the cornea. But the molecular structure of water is much like the cornea's, so the corneas of fish and deep-sea mammals have become flattened and have no light-bending function; they simply keep debris out of the eye. However, land creatures, lacking a water environment to do the initial refracting, require a curved cornea. The lens is a fine-tuner for terrestrial animals; the cornea does most of the work.

It took a great deal of time for nature to evolve a curved cornea that could bend light. Today's amphibians have normal sight on land during adulthood, but at different junctures in their lives they must return to the water to breed or to escape predators or to find food. With their curved corneas, they have become farsighted in water. "Double life" or no, they cannot have it both ways—they can't see well in both media. It is not until we encounter the extraordinary eye of a particular seabird that we will discover a creature that sees as well underwater as on land.

The First Amphibians

Amphibians are divided into three classes, the anurans (frogs and toads), the urodeles (newts and salamanders) and the caecilians, though the last are the least interesting visually. But all amphibians are descended from an ancient, extinct fish called a crossopterygian. The amphibians' descent from fish is evident in the similarity of their photoreceptors to those of two ancient fish that still swim in the oceans and rivers of the world, the holosteans and the dipnoans (lungfish). But specific

visual characteristics reinforce science's belief that yet another fish was the ancestor of the modern teleost, or bony, fish.

That ancient crossopterygian fish had eyes with pupils able to widen or contract in response to a decrease or increase in light, while the ancestor of teleost fish did not. Consequently, fish are dependent on the internal movement of screening pigment to protect them from glare; since this movement is slow, they are extremely vulnerable to sudden changes in light intensity. But the amphibian was the first vertebrate to have a neural mechanism that required pupillary contraction. Moreover, the visual legacy of that crossopterygian fish also made possible another change in the eye. Since the ciliary muscles of the iris regulate the amount of light entering the eye, the lens fell back closer to the retina, where its function became to change focus from near to far vision or vice versa.

Visual Aspects of Metamorphosis

When hatched in water, the tadpole bears very little resemblance to the adult frog. While adult toads and frogs are essentially visual creatures, image formation is apparently of very limited importance at the larval stage. Some tadpoles feed in the dark and eat dead insects or algae.

Despite the tadpole's visual limitations, nature has made every possible effort to give these creatures a chance to see. The visual pigment (porphyropsin) that absorbs the photons is the same type found in freshwater fish. Based on Vitamin A_2, porphyropsin is more sensitive to the longer wavelengths of light that penetrate freshwater ponds. Its wavelength maximum is 522nm, which means that, while tadpoles may not see in color, they are certainly aware of shades of light and dark and perhaps even the shape of objects and fish in their pond.

By the time adulthood has been reached and the frog has emerged from the pond, a visual metamorphosis has taken place: The visual pigment has become rhodopsin, based on Vitamin A_1, with a wavelength maximum of about 500nm, which means that it is more sensitive to shorter wavelengths. We know that some frogs even exhibit a distinct preference for the color blue.

Tadpoles respond to light even if their eyes are nonfunctional. They have pineal and parietal glands on the tops of their heads that contain rodlike photoreceptors. While not eyes in the true sense, those organs do play an important role in the hormonal changes that occur as the tadpole metamorphoses into an adult frog or toad.

One of the more interesting aquatic amphibians, the Mexican water salamander known as the axolotl (the name translates from the Aztec as "water monster"), appears to remain in an immature stage for its entire life. When scientists inject them with hormones, they develop into terrestrial salamanders. As one would expect, they have normal sight in water but become extremely nearsighted on land.

The Anatomy of The Amphibian Eye

The eyes of frogs and toads are large and spherical and protrude from either side of the head. They have been described as periscopic, and they give these creatures a 360-degree panoramic view of their environment. The orbit of the eye is so large, in fact, that it extends down into the pharynx. Two muscles, the retractor bulbi, help the eyes perform a most unusual function; by retracting the eyes into the pharynx, the muscles hold down a struggling prey and help force it down the frog's throat. This is their only eye movement; the eyes do not move in the sockets.

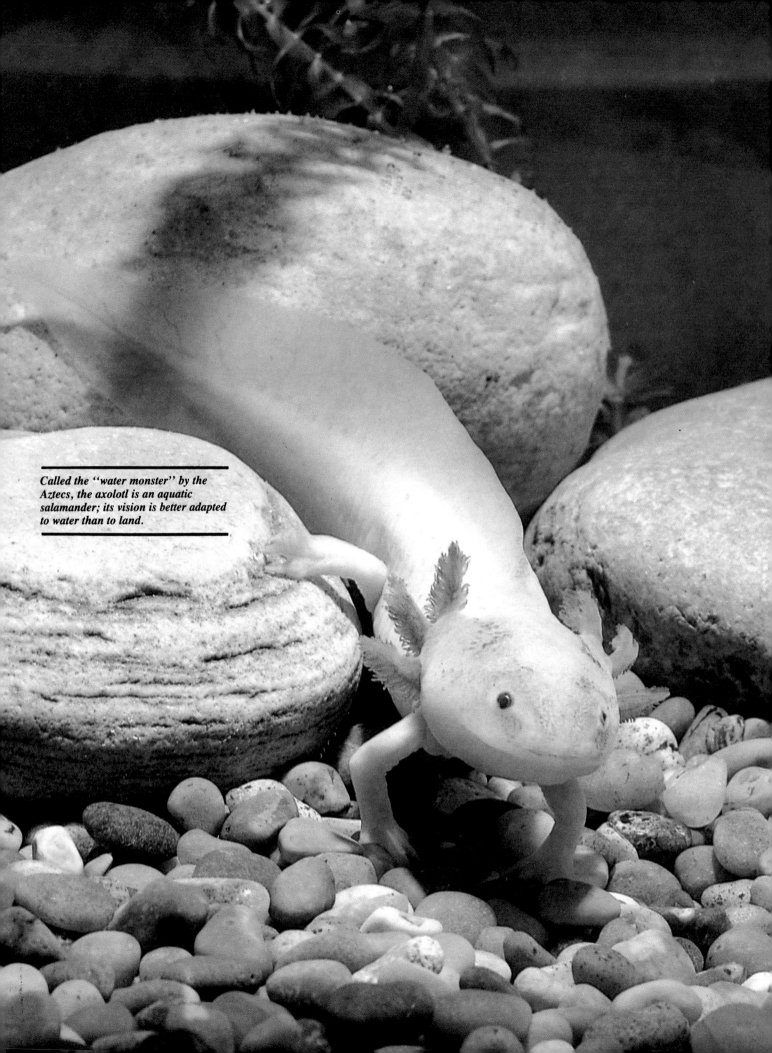

Called the "water monster" by the Aztecs, the axolotl is an aquatic salamander; its vision is better adapted to water than to land.

The lens of the frog or toad is spherical (like that of the fish) in the tadpole stage but flattens out and moves to the rear in adulthood. Accommodation for near and far vision resembles the shark's; a muscle moves the lens forward in sort of a pendular movement rather than changing the shape of the lens.

Frogs and some toads have beautiful eyes. Their irises are packed with colored melanophores that give different species their characteristic color—golden yellow in the North American bullfrog, blue in the Asian flying frog, and red in the Costa Rican tree frog, to name a few. When dilated, the pupils are round, but when contracted, they assume a variety of forms: pear-shaped, heart-shaped, etc., depending on the species. A pupillary stripe the color of the frog's skin extends the length of the eye. While the pupils contract in response to light, the ciliary muscles are very weak, and a great deal of light is required for this change to occur.

Since the amphibian no longer had environmental water to cleanse the eye, it was the first creature to develop lachrymal glands that secrete tears. Amphibians also have harderian glands that secrete an oily lubricant, something that is fairly common to creatures who spend any time in the water; the oil is spread over the eye by the movement of the lower eyelid. Terrestrial amphibians have both lower and upper eyelids, but these develop only in adulthood.

The Eye of Newts and Salamanders (the Urodeles)

Why do witches always add the eye of a newt to their potions? Certainly it is inferior to the eye of the toad or the frog. Besides, it is mainly their tails that distinguish the urodeles from other amphibians. Most newts and salamanders live under rocks where complex image formation isn't necessary. One distinctive feature of the urodelian eye is the comparatively large lens. The sclera (the tissue that surrounds the eye) and the choroid layer (which nourishes the retina) are crude in design and shape. The cells are comparatively fibrous and disorganized, a sign of a more primitive, less-evolved being. The photoreceptors of the retina are larger and fewer than those of the anuran retina, which means that the picture of the world seen by the newt or salamander lacks fine detail. It is life in broad strokes with little refinement. Yet the size of the rod photoreceptors in the tiger salamander are far larger than most other creatures'—100 microns, where the norm for rods is 20 microns and cones can be as small as 2 or 3 microns.

Yet nature has tried some very interesting experiments with the eyes of certain salamanders and newts native to Japan. In the first place, the Japanese salamander is the largest urodele in the world, measuring up to five feet in length—quite a difference from those we are used to. It must have been a challenge for nature to figure a way to feed the cornea. All parts of the body require nourishment, usually carried through a net-

The eyes of frogs are filled with brilliant iridocytes that color their eyes. Pupils are found in a wide variety of shapes: heart, pear, round, oval, etc., and it is possible to identify the type of frog from the shape of the pupil. Shown here are the great river frog (left) and the horned frog.

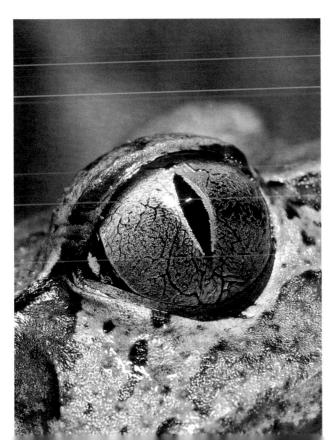

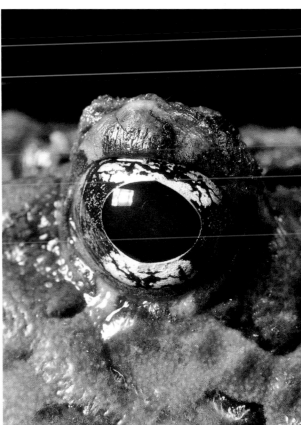

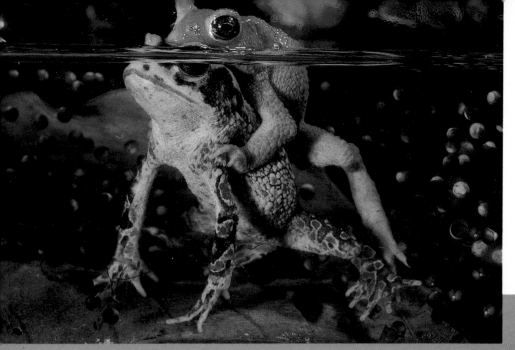

The golden toads of Costa Rica cannot call to their mates like other frogs or toads and must rely instead on their brilliant coloration.

▼

Arrowpoison frogs, like other South American poisonous amphibians, are brilliantly colored to warn away would-be predators.

work of blood vessels of gradually decreasing size. But if blood vessels are placed in the cornea itself, how can the animal see? But this is exactly what happened in the case of all Japanese urodeles: They have a vascular network throughout the cornea. It must be something like looking through a grill. This natural experiment was discontinued elsewhere in the world, however, and most corneas are clear, like ours, and are nourished by the aqueous humor, the jellylike layer that is right next to the cornea.

As in other amphibians, the pupil of the urodelian eye is round when dilated and the iris is brilliantly colored, some with metallic flecks or green-and-brown banding.

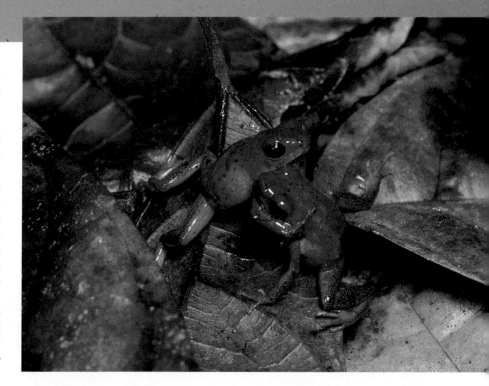

Color Vision in Amphibians

Most amphibians have some color vision, though it may be restricted to narrow bands of the spectrum. Some amphibians may have their color vision affected by rods as well as cones; in fact, one rod, the so-called green rod, may play an important role.

There are four types of photoreceptors in the amphibian retina. The first is called the violet rod. It is plump, contains rhodopsin, yet has some characteristics of a cone; its outer segment is very large and in contact with the external membrane. The so-called green rod is found only in amphibians. The outer, smaller segment lacks rhodopsin, and the nucleus is very deep at the bottom of a long, slim stalk. Its structure seems to be midway between that of a cone and an ordinary red rod. The single cones resemble those of holostean and Dipnoi fish, and diurnal types have a yellow oil droplet. The double cones have no oil droplets, with one larger and one smaller accessory segment.

Most European salamanders are themselves brightly colored, which is generally a clue to whether creatures themselves can also see in color. Some of them even appear to favor brightly colored backgrounds. Behavioral tests indicate an ability to distinguish

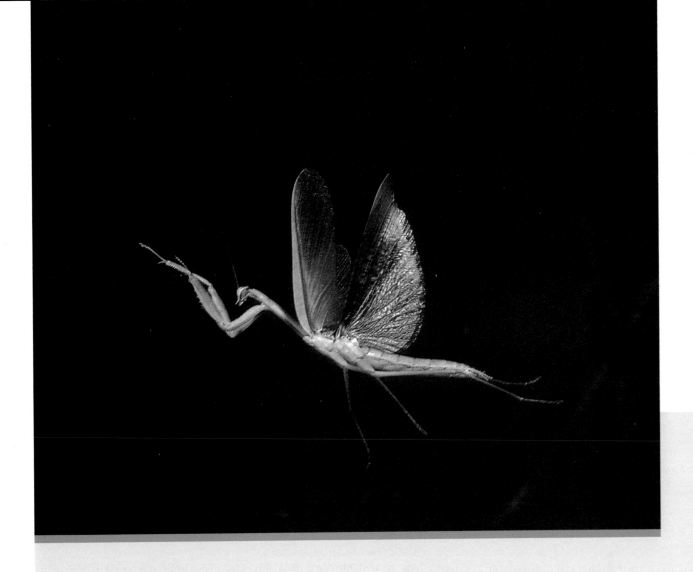

orange, yellow and possibly even red and green.

Frogs show a distinct preference for the color blue. So marked is this preference that if green is added to the blue, the frog will actively avoid the spot. Now, it is easy to deduce that escape for most amphibians means a jump in the (blue) water, but no one seems to be able to explain the avoidance of the color green. Also, this is not true of all amphibians. *Salamandra salamandra* not only likes green, but is especially responsive to greens that fall at about 570nm. Testing has shown that some amphibians are what is called *photonegative;* that is, they show absolutely no response to color whatsoever—though it is difficult to believe that any of these creatures is totally color blind.

Nocturnal Amphibians

Many toads are nocturnal. With their delicate skin, what better way to avoid desiccation? Unlike diurnal frogs, nocturnal toads have no oil droplets in the cones of their retinas. For a long time it was assumed that they had no color vision, but that bane of the vision scientist, a boring test, proved to be the culprit: Toads will simply not respond if the same test is repeated over and over again.

While neither frogs nor toads have tapeta, their visual cells do contain a fair amount of guanine, the reflective material found in the scales and tapeta of fish. It makes their eyes appear to glow.

▲

This is the way a moving praying mantis may appear to a frog. Many scientists believe that the frog's eye can detect only motion and cannot see stationary objects at all.

Visual Acuity in Frogs and Toads

Frogs and toads are essentially visual creatures, more so than newts and salamanders, though even their range of vision is not great. We know that they can recognize a variety of shapes. For instance, those that have had the misfortune to eat a bee or wasp avoid them thereafter and even stay away from the robber fly, which mimics the bee.

Most frogs and toads have a range around their body known as *the snapping zone*. Any insect or worm that ventures into this area will be snapped at. The snapping zone of the toad is more limited than the frog's, though apparently this is because of the former's smaller body size.

Frogs and toads can recognize their mates visually when they are about seven or eight inches away. They use landmarks to recognize their territory as well. Some frogs may even be able to orient themselves by the stars: For example, frogs that have been captured during the day then released at night have found their way back to the area of their capture.

The upper part of frogs' and toads' visual field is apparently important in avoiding predators, while the lower part is concerned mainly with searching out surfaces on which the animal can jump. As we know, the frog prefers to jump on a blue surface. Also, in seeking escape, tests show, it chooses an opening with horizontal lines rather than vertical ones.

Vision and Behavior

It would be an exaggeration to say that a frog's eye does most of the animal's thinking, but the eye of the amphibian *is* coded to respond to certain visual stimuli. This is a creature with a very simple brain, and it responds almost immediately to what it sees. The two visual centers of the brain, the optic tectum and the thalamus, operate separately, with the optic tectum important to prey-catching and the thalamus controlling avoidance of predators. While there is no neocortex to store memories, there is apparently enough room in the thalamus for amphibians to remember the shape and color of a bee or wasp or other insect that has caused pain.

Eyes with receptor cells that trigger behavior are found in creatures with less-developed nervous systems; obviously their behavior is much less flexible than ours.

The frog has four types of ganglion cells, one of which is sometimes playfully described as a "bug detector" but is known more scientifically as a moving-edge detector; there are also a net-convexity detector, a net-dimming detector, and a sustained-contrast cell. Much emphasis has been placed on frogs' ability to detect movement. They leap from a lily pad, throw out their sticky tongue, and catch an insect on the wing. For a creature with only four types of receptor cells, that's pretty good coordinated movement. But some scientists believe that frogs detect movement so well because they cannot see anything that is stationary. Since the background does not interfere, the moving object stands out. Put a frog in a cage with dead, motionless worms, and it may well starve to death. However, it is known that some kinds of frogs are better at pattern formation than others; for example, ranid frogs see better than hylan frogs.

The eye of the frog is such an excellent motion detector that the manmade electric eye is actually based on its structure. The ability of a frog to capture a moving insect is limited by its range of vision. Within the snapping range, it probably sees best when a creature is moving quickly since the background does tend to blur.

No doubt, the image that the frog or toad has of its world cannot be compared with the detail and color perceived by the human eye. It has to be a crude picture compared with our own. But if you've ever been bitten by an insect, tried to swat it, and missed, you might have deduced that the frog's eye does have certain advantages: Thought takes time.

Another major advantage of the amphibian eye is its ability to regenerate damaged portions of the visual system. A newt can replace a dam-

aged eye within the year. It simply grows back. A frog whose optic nerves have been severed can regenerate them within months. In this case, the penalty that more complex animals pay for their developed irreplaceable visual system is high indeed.

9 Reptiles

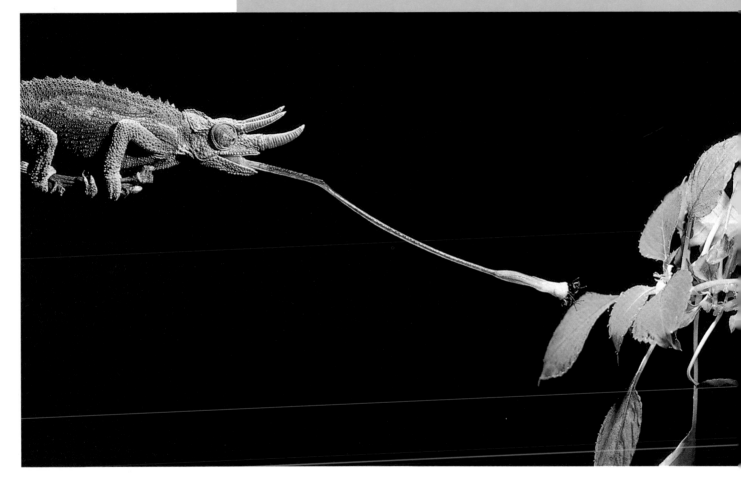

It is difficult to imagine that the reptiles of today are descended from the enormous creatures whose bones can be seen in museums, their sightless orbits staring down from splendid heights. We can only glean some idea of their visual acuity from the reptiles of our own time, some of whom have evolved remarkable visual devices in the 65 million years or so since the beginning of their decline as the dominant form of life on earth. For instance, certain snakes have developed infrared sensors that enable them to of warm-blooded creatures as well as

to form a more conventional visual image. Other reptiles, such as crocodiles and alligators, have become nocturnal. Nocturnality was unknown to the giant reptiles; since they could not generate their own body heat they became torpid at night. It is also possible that the dinosaurs, like some of their cone-rich descendants, the turtles, were practically blind after dark.

There are few existing reptilian species: the chelonians, or turtles, terrapins and tortoises; the rhynchocephalians, who have one living member, a nocturnal lizard called the

▲

When both of the Jackson's three-horned chameleon's eyes focus together, this fly will have little chance of escape. But experiments have shown that even with one eye closed, the chameleon is capable of using visual clues such as distance, interposition and gradient to capture its prey.

sphenodon who is found only in New Zealand and whose outstanding visual characteristic is a third eye in the middle of its head; the lacertilians, or lizards; and the ophidians, or snakes,

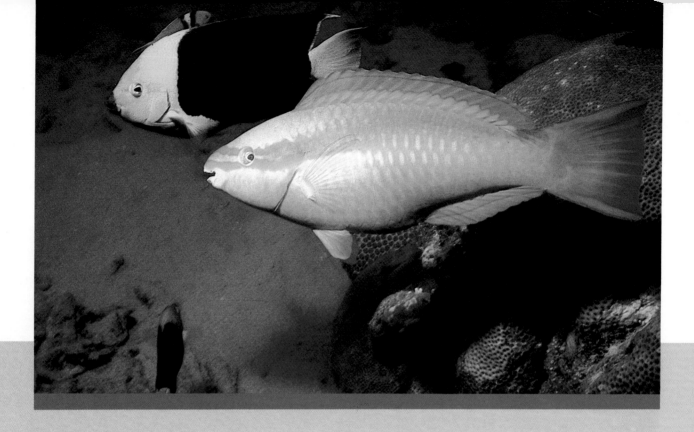

who are descended from lizards who sought refuge by fleeing underground and gradually lost their limbs in the process. And yet the ingenuity of nature never fails to amaze: When snakes returned above ground, some of them had learned to "see" in the dark; but what they "see" is heat radiated by the warm body of their prey.

Changes in vision do not occur in isolation; they are often in response to a change in habitat. In the case of the amphibian, who developed the ability to breathe on land, the eye adapted a curved cornea better suited to a dry environment (see chapter 8). Deep-sea fish swam to the depths of the ocean for safety; the eye also adapted. Moreover, these adaptations frequently have repercussions further down the evolutionary line.

For example, the reptile was the first creature to accommodate for near and far vision by changing the shape of its lens and making it more convex or concave, using muscles that don't even exist in the amphibian or fish. These creatures do not see well at a distance, and neither does the reptile,

but this particular modification would one day give many birds and mammals an incredible range of focus.

Now that the primary burden of focusing light on the retina had fallen to the cornea, a change that began with the amphibian, the lens fell back behind the iris, and the reptiles' eyes became motile. For the first time, a creature could follow an object by moving its eyes in their sockets. The chameleon carries this ability to extremes; it can look in two different directions at once.

Depth perception also improved; a new muscle, the ventral transversalis, swung the lens toward the nose, allowing for improved eye convergence and marking the beginning of binocular vision. Annular muscles attached to either side of the lens improved the reptile's ability to scan the horizon.

These are the basic improvements made in the reptilian eye. No doubt it is a better terrestrial eye than is the amphibian's. One indication is that the reptile preys on the amphibian and not vice versa. Each succeed-

▲ ▲
Only the eyes of the sea turtle and some birds contain red oil droplets in the individual photoreceptors. These block the shorter wavelengths, thus shifting color vision to the longer wavelengths. Here are two fish as they would appear to us and as they might appear to a sea turtle.

ing species appears to survive by preying on creatures who are less evolved, unless the latter are able to hide themselves till a new adaptation is made in their own structure. For instance, we know that mammals survived the age of the dominant reptiles by escaping into nocturnality. Is it possible that another creature is evolving right under our noses that will one day replace us as the dominant species on this planet? There are already animals who make wider use of the electromagnetic spectrum than we do—most insects and snakes with infrared vision—and while we are so proud of our brains, whales and dolphins have a larger neocortex. Perhaps it is only a matter of time. . . .

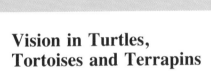

Vision in Turtles, Tortoises and Terrapins

They are the most ancient of living reptiles, their soft bodies encased in a hard protective shell. While never noted for their speed, the *Cheloniidae,* or sea turtles, at least have their great weight supported by water and move through the seas with flippers instead of feet. The land tortoise, however, must make its way on foot. The terrapin is a North American freshwater turtle distinguished by its webbed feet.

At one time it was thought that the turtle had a pure cone retina; we now know that there are a very few rods mixed in, certainly not enough to change the distinguishing characteristics of almost pure cone vision. These creatures see very poorly in dim light and are virtually blind at night. Dim light conditions abound in the ocean, though sea turtles stick to surface waters and are not known for deep diving; the reason is obvious. Pure rod retinas are more common in the animal kingdom than almost pure cone

retinas, though most vision authorities believe that the cone developed first and the rod evolved later when a variety of animals sought safety in the dark of night. The almost pure cone retina pops up in unusual places: also in the squirrel and prairie dog, for instance, which are related. Perhaps it can be explained by the inability of the earliest reptiles to create their own body heat; thus limited to daylight activity, there was no reason for them to develop rods.

The eyes of all chelonians are very small. But from here on in, let's simply call them turtles. The lens is flat or more like an ellipse in land turtles and spherical in the marine; it is also the softest and most malleable of any vertebrate lens, though only the land turtle changes its shape for near and far vision. The annular pads in turtles are quite weak, which means they spend very little time scanning the horizon. Their interests are obviously more aroused at close quarters, though some can catch insects on the fly, and domesticated turtles have been known to recognize their

masters at a distance of 50 meters.

Turtles that divide their time between life on land and in the water are forced to contend with the same problems as are their amphibian precursors. *Chelonia mydas* is normally sighted in water but becomes myopic on land. *Gopherus polyphemus* is farsighted in air and becomes even more farsighted in water. Very few have good vision in both media; *Clemmys insculpta* and the freshwater turtle *Pseudemys* appear to be rare exceptions, though even their sight can never be perfect in both.

The cones of turtles are distinguished by the presence of red, yellow and orange oil droplets that act as a filtration system, blocking light of certain wavelengths and allowing others to pass. Only turtles and birds possess red oil droplets. The droplets are positioned in a portion of the retina through which light must pass before reaching the visual pigment. Since the prime function of oil droplets is to block shorter wavelengths, color vision in turtles would be best in the longer wavelengths: yellows, or-

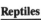

anges and reds. Greens, blues and violets must be difficult for them to distinguish. Why do only birds and turtles have red oil droplets?

First, red droplets are generally found in the pigeon and certain types of seabird that must frequently fly great distances through fog and bad weather and locate fish swimming beneath the water despite the glare of the water's surface. The red droplets act as filters to increase contrast. Sea turtles are also great navigators and must similarly voyage through thousands of miles of ocean to return to a particular spot on land to lay their eggs. They also suffer from the glare of down-welling light; not only do the

droplets improve contrast, but they must also be protection against dazzlement, or blinding from too much light. Here the turtle is particularly vulnerable, since it is the only reptile whose pupils do not contract, although it does have eyelids.

Normally creatures that live in seas or oceans are more sensitive to shorter-wavelength light (blue) while those that live in fresh water respond to longer wavelengths (red). Red oil droplets in sea turtles make them an exception to this rule. Since sea turtles are known to remain in shallower waters still illuminated by longer-wavelength light, the visual image presented to their eyes will be char-

acterized by a desaturization of the surrounding blue water; colored objects such as coral, anemones and fish should therefore stand out. The visual pigment of sea turtles is, as usual, made up of chromoproteins based on rhodopsin while that of freshwater turtles is based on porphyropsin.

Turtles retain the ability to retract their eyes into their heads when danger presents itself; they do not appear to use this technique as does the frog or toad, for whom it is sort of a digestive aid (see chapter 8). Of the two eyelids, the lower is the mobile one. Occasionally the lower lid is transparent, but the turtle also has a semi-opaque nictitating membrane

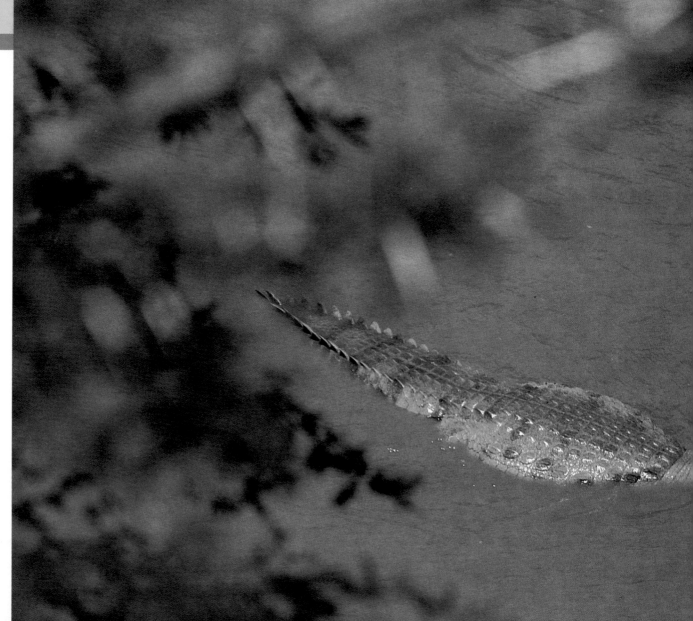

that sweeps over the eye to clean and protect it.

Whether it is to escape the dazzlement of too much sunlight reflected by the beach or to protect her vulnerable eyes from blowing bits of sand or debris, the female sea turtle is known to emerge from the water to lay her eggs with her eyes tightly shut. They do not open until she is back in the water. The most interesting question of all is how she finds her way to this same spot year after year in the first place. It is a formidable piece of navigation, similar in many respects to the legendary navigational experiences of pigeons and seabirds.

Some believe that vision does not play a role in this journey; after all, eels return to the same island, Anguilla in the British West Indies, and salmon return to their streams supposedly without the aid of vision. We know that the position of the sun plays a role in the navigational abilities of bees, but they have the capacity to perceive polarized light, something that until recently was not thought to apply to vertebrates. But if a new theory is correct, birds and possibly even turtles may share this capacity (see chapter 10). This would mean that despite glare or even dim light conditions, the turtle would be able to navigate by the position of the sun.

Turtles subjected to a variety of tests have been able to identify a wide variety of objects and shapes. They can distinguish between horizontal and vertical lines and make their way through a maze successfully. (But what's a maze when one can navigate thousands of miles through an ocean?) They can identify circles and triangles, will avoid objects associated with electric shock, and will press levers that reward them with food. Such behavior is impressive, considering that they are the most ancient living reptile. Speed obviously isn't everything.

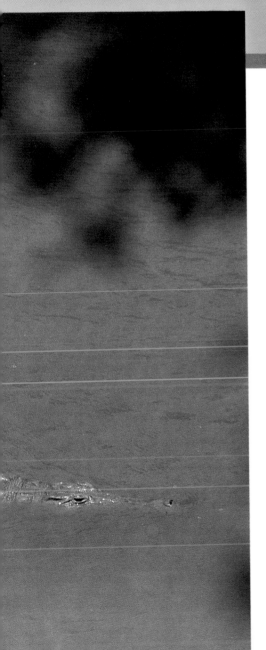

Vision in Crocodiles and Alligators (the Crocodilians)

They float through the water or wait in shallow depths with only their eyes and snout showing slightly above the water. Their eyes are encased in large, spherical bony structures that protrude from the top of either side of the head, so that they can discover prey above the water while the rest of their bodies remain hidden.

These largest of the reptiles (20 to 30 feet long) are nocturnal. Should a light strike the eyes, they glow with the color of their visual pigment—red in the alligator, more of an orange in the crocodile. Only rods are present in their retinas, in contrast to the cone-rich retinas of turtles.

◀

As the Nile crocodile lies in wait, sometimes only the eyes and snout are visible.

While sluggish on land, alligators and crocodiles can move through the water with great speed to catch their unlucky prey, perhaps a water buffalo or wild pig that has come to drink. They are not discriminating eaters, as we know from too many bad movies. And while they spend much of their time in the water, their vision is better out of it. It's thought that their vision isn't very acute even in air, but this may be premature since they are one of the few animals with predominantly rod retinas to have fovea, i.e., a small, round area of the retina that contains large numbers of densely packed photoreceptors, making possible that perception of fine detail. (The eye of the crocodile or alligator is not very mobile, however, and this may be one of the reasons for its limited vision.)

Unlike those of the turtle, the pupils of the crocodilian contract, reacting to light (and human-administered drugs). Like other nocturnal animals, they have a slit pupil. But when contracted, it forms what is called a stenopeic pupil, a feature shared with only a few other creatures—sea snakes, nocturnal geckoes, and seals, all of whom spend a lot of time in the water. Each stenopeic pupil contracts to form two small holes so small they have been compared to a pinhole camera. This gives the creature better focus over a great depth of field without any lens accommodation; however, they require a great deal of light to form an image. Then why would a nocturnal creature have a stenopeic pupil?

First, there are times when a crocodilian must be active during the day; the stenopeic pupil protects its sensitive rods from temporary blinding from too much light. Second, while crocodilians are able to change the shape of their lens for near and far vision, the ciliary muscles are very weak; the stenopeic pupil, however, allows for better focus over great distance. One can almost think of it as an accessory lens.

Crocodilians have an upper mobile eyelid and a well-developed nictitating membrane; the latter is so transparent that it is possible to see the iris right through it. Both lachrymal and harderian glands bathe and cleanse the eye, though for some reason it has become common to describe crocodile tears as false tears. What, people ask, could a crocodilian have to cry about, with its savage jaws and small eyes? And yet I carry within me the image of an alligator described by a photographer who took many of the pictures in this book. On one of his trips to Africa, natives took him to a cave where an alligator had been sleeping for two years, avoiding the terrible drought that had stricken most of North Africa. The animal's eyes were shut tightly and it scarcely breathed. It had no moisture left for tears, but it was surviving . . . waiting for the rains to come.

Vision in Lizards

There are so many different types of lizards, geckoes, Gila monsters, glass snakes, slowworms, skinks, iguanas. . . . Like their relatives, the chelonians and the crocodilians, they have adapted to life on land. Most of them have skin that does not have to be bathed in water, and their eggs have coverings that let them survive on land.

Like other reptiles, lizards adapt for near and far vision by squeezing or stretching the lens with both ciliary muscles and annular pads. The eyeball is spherical, and each lizard eye has a brightly colored iris with a brilliant sheen due to a layer of guanine iridocytes.

To protect the eye from excessive light, the pupils contract. The nocturnal gecko has a slit pupil that becomes a stenopeic pupil like that of the crocodilian, but the pupil of the diurnal gecko is round. The photoreceptors are also protected by the movement of visual pigment, though this is far less important for the gecko than for fish.

One of the features that distinguishes the eye of the lizard from that of other creatures, including other reptiles, is an extension of the choroid body called the conus papillaris, which nourishes the lizard's cornea. It projects right into the vitreous humor, even though its presence must impede the flow of photons through the retina. Perhaps for that very reason, it has been sacrificed in other creatures.

The eyes of the chameleon are the most motile of any lizard; they are able to look in two different directions at the same time. Sometimes they even look in front and back simultaneously. Whether the chameleon's tiny

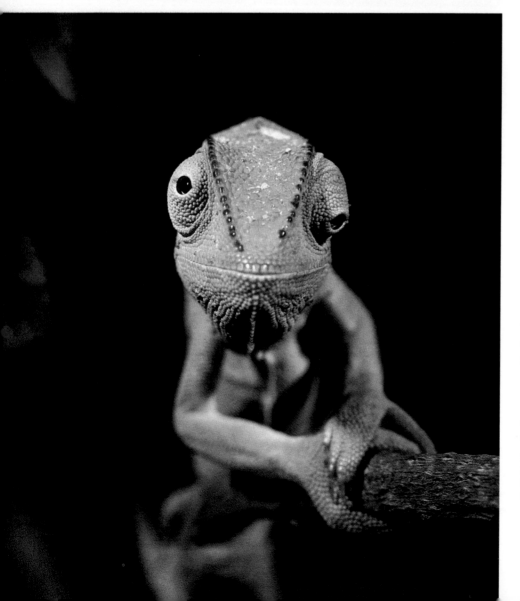

◀

While the vision of the Senegalese chameleon is limited by its barrel-like skin covering, the eyes are so mobile that this creature can look in two directions at once.

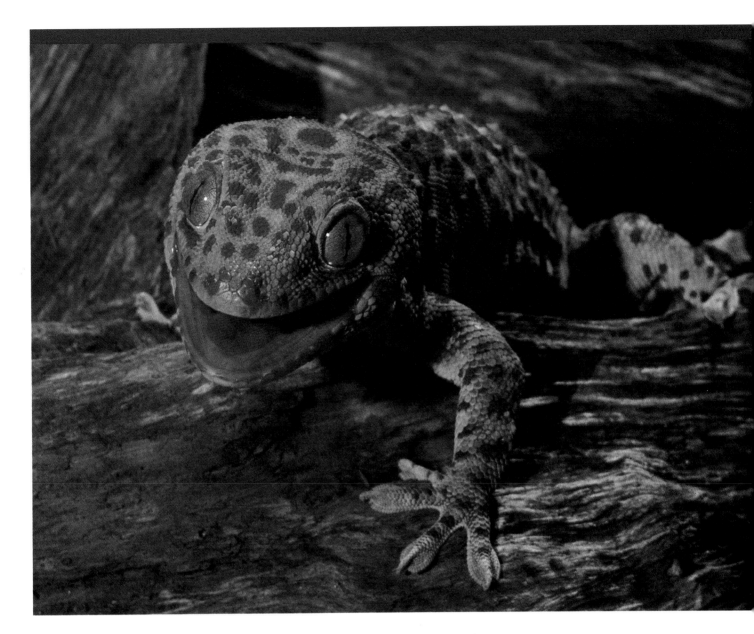

brain suppresses one or the other image or has some sort of split-screen mechanism to compare both pictures is not known. But they can also bring both eyes together to converge on one spot. It is possible that until both eyes converge, they don't form an integrated image but are only aware of movement. Perhaps, then, one could compare their split vision to our own peripheral vision: We aren't really aware of what happens on the periphery of our vision until a movement there causes us to focus on that spot. However, the binocular vision of the chameleon is limited by the great round folds of skin that encase the eyes and limit its visual field. Holding two telescopes up to our eyes might give us some idea of what the world looks like to the chameleon—a strange sort of tunnel vision in two directions at once.

While binocular vision begins with the convergence of two eyes on the same object, tests have shown that lizards use monocular cues as much as visual overlap to trap insects on the fly. When scientists cover one of its eyes, Jackson's chameleon's long, sticky tongue still is able to trap insects and jerk them back into its mouth. While binocular vision enhances depth perception, nature has not left the one-eyed without resources.

Closing one's eyes and shutting out the world can be soothing for

Like the crocodile, the Tokay gecko has a stenopaic pupil, clearly visible in this picture. The pupil, which shuts down to two tiny holes, is normally found in creatures that spend a good deal of time in water.

human beings. We have only one lid that is mobile; lizards are fortunate enough to have two. But many lizards have a transparent lid, enabling them to protect their eyes during a sandstorm and still see something of the world. The West Indian *Anolis* lizard has a transparent lower lid. The skink Ablepharus has two lids that have fused to become a single transparent spectacle.

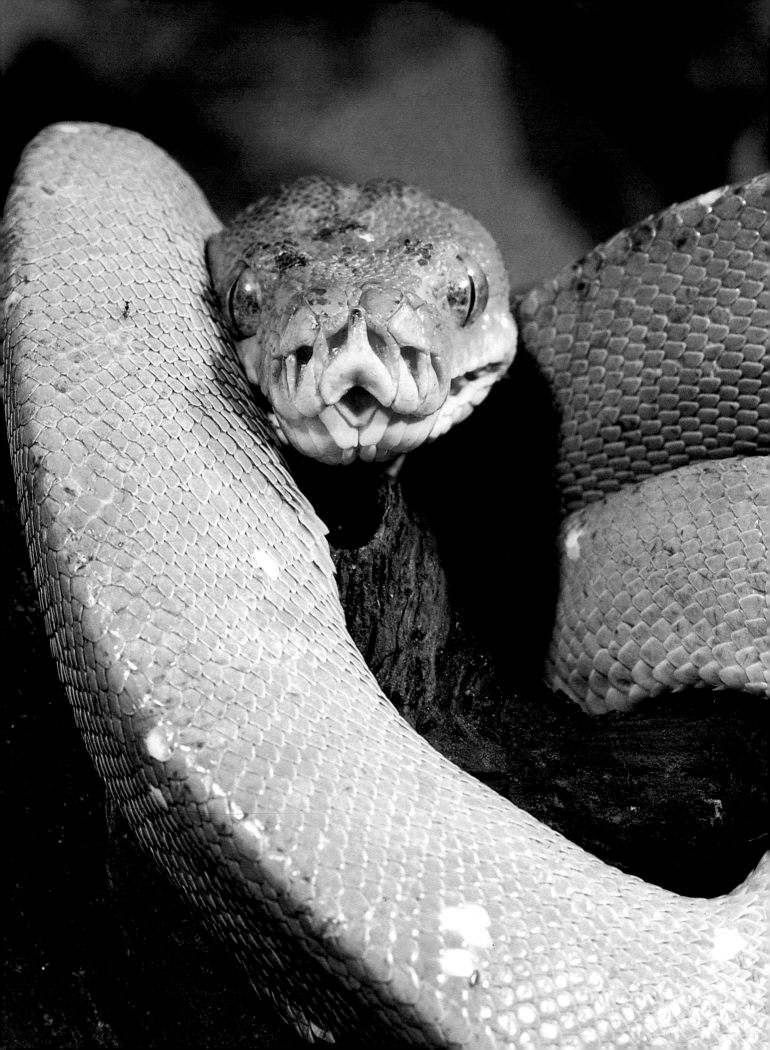

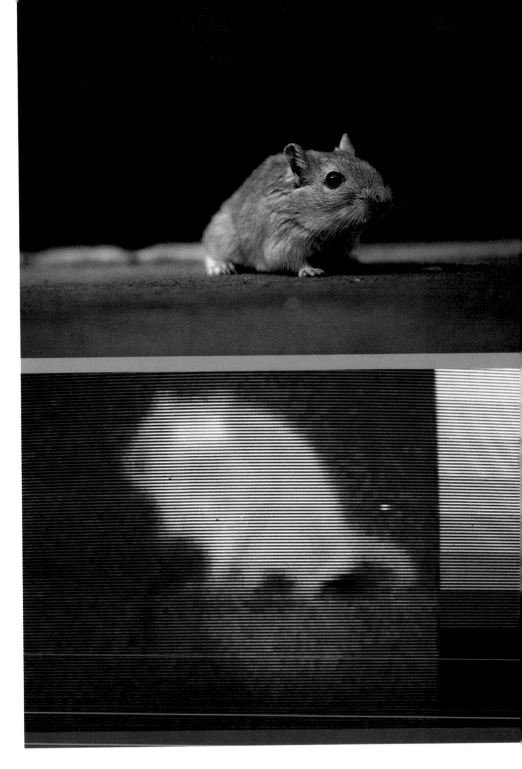

Cave-dwelling lizards have eyes surrounded by a black circle, which absorbs light and heat when they leave the protection of their dark surroundings. They share this natural protection with the cheetah, which is the only diurnal predatory cat (football players have to paint theirs on).

The vision of most lizards is excellent, and only the limbless among them are truly limited in optical image formation. (We speak here primarily of creatures like the skink and not snakes, which must be considered on their own terms.) Many lizards have photoreceptors that are responsive to ultraviolet light. Diurnal lizards have a fovea, perhaps the first one evolved. The fovea is most developed in the chameleon, whose cones are longer and more concentrated than our own (756,000 compared to 200,000 per sq mm). The tree-living *Anolis* lizard has two foveas, one in the central part of the retina and the other in the periphery, thus supporting the general rule that arboreal creatures have better vision than their ground-dwelling relatives.

Vision in Snakes

Snakes provoke a revulsion in many people that is not matched by turtles or even crocodilians. However, some snakes have evolved an eye unique among all other eyes on earth as not only a detector of light frequency but as a detector of energy as well. A dim bulb appears brighter in the dark than in daylight because the eye adapts, not because the bulb gives off more energy. But the eye of a pit viper or a boid (pronounced *bo-id*), would not make the same mistake: The bulb would appear the same to it regardless of the brightness of the background.

At some point, all snakes burrowed under ground. Proof of a long period of life under the earth is found in the loss of colored oil droplets in the individual photoreceptors, which at the very least protect the eye from ultraviolet damage and chromatic aberration (a blurring of the visual image, which will be discussed in detail further on). Nature replaced the droplets with one yellow filter which

One photograph of this gerbil was taken normally and the other with an AGA thermographic camera, which records infrared radiation not normally visible to our own eyes but which is visible to both boids and pit vipers, such as rattlers. This gerbil would be visible to those snakes even in pitch dark.

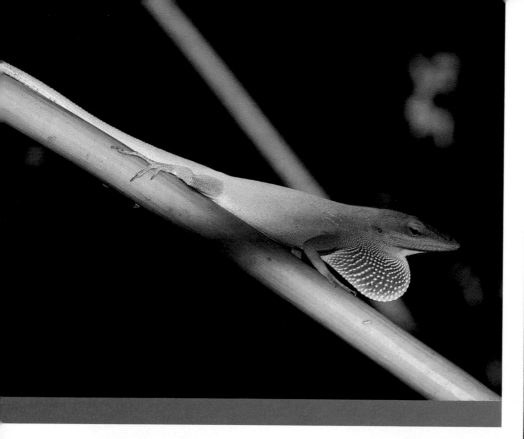

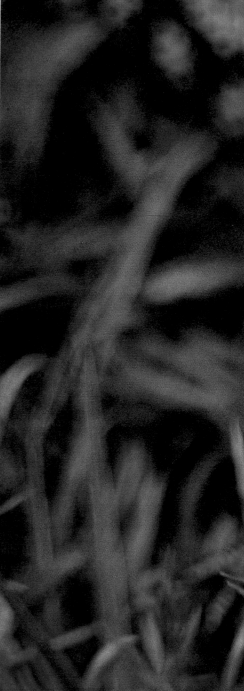

▲

The anole lizard's lower lid has become a transparent spectacle; the animal can see even with its eyes closed, which helps it during sandstorms.

completely fills the lens and thus absorbs ultraviolet and near-ultraviolet light. This filter is very much like our own, as our forebears also lost their oil droplets at a time when nature had adopted a new method of filtration.

Most snakes eventually became diurnal, with mixed rod and cone vision and the capacity to see in color. Diurnal snakes have round pupils, and nocturnal snakes have slit pupils. Despite their nocturnality, the feared krait of Asia and the fer-de-lance of South America did not develop infrared vision. The boids and the pit vipers did (Pythons, boa constrictors, water moccasins, copperheads and rattlesnakes). These are the ones who can truly see in the dark, despite the fact that they are basically diurnal. The combination of infrared and normal vision gives them an incalculable advantage in the struggle to survive. It is as if these creatures have two separate, overlapping visual systems,

improving the overall picture in the way that humans can use both sound and sight to locate an object.

Infrared vision developed from a completely different part of the snake's nervous system, the trigeminal nerve, used in humans to convey touch, pain and warmth. (Remember that the eye of the invertebrate developed from skin while only the vertebrate eye developed from a part of the brain.) The python of Southeast Asia has 13 pairs of reticulated pits around its mouth, while most vipers have theirs under the eyes. These pits function much like a pinhole camera, conveying a sense of distance as well as an image. Combined heat and visual images are sent via the optic nerve, which in snakes has the most connections, to a region of their brain called the optic tectum. Here the images are combined by tectal cells that respond to both or to one or the other. (The entire optic tectum has become an area of the mammalian brain called the superior colliculus, which is the main center for processing an image in space; and in monkeys, the tectum initiates and controls looking.) We know that the combination of color and form vastly improves a creature's ability to locate an object in space. There is no doubt that the overlapping heat and visual images have somewhat the same effect in the vision of snakes. One wonders where nature will apply this technique again.

According to experiments conducted by Gamow and Harris, a boa constrictor will respond to diffuse light from infrared radiation from a carbon dioxide laser in 35 milliseconds, while a man-made instrument requires nearly a minute to make the same measurement. The adjacent thermogram of a mouse should give you some idea of the quality of the heat image that overlays the snake's visual image.

And yet the normal vision of snakes is good, despite popular myths to the contrary. The cobra is the most visually oriented snake, relying mainly on vision rather than on its sense of smell, as do other snakes. When a cobra or python weaves back and forth in front of you, it's just putting you

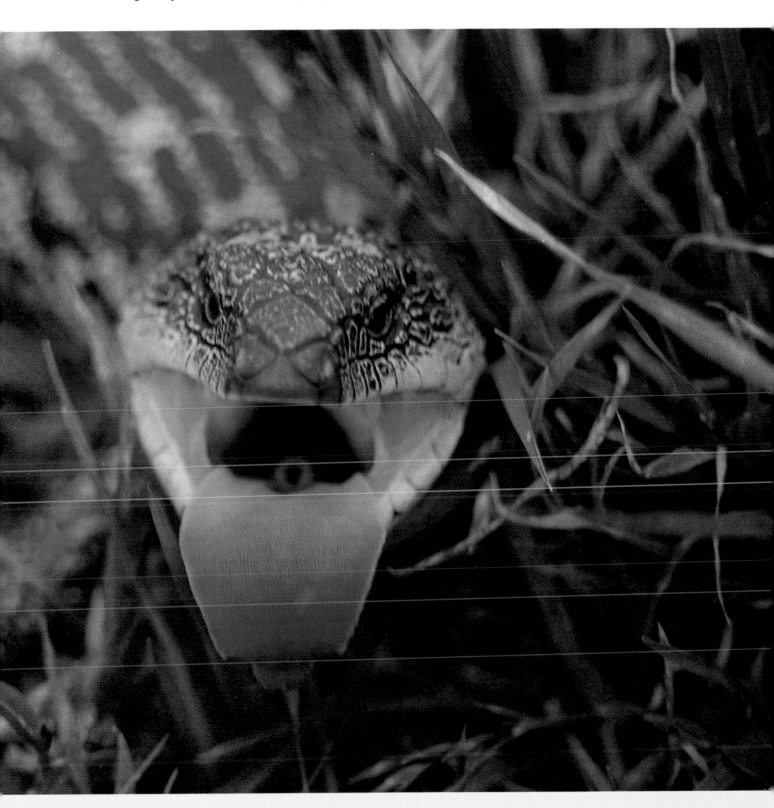

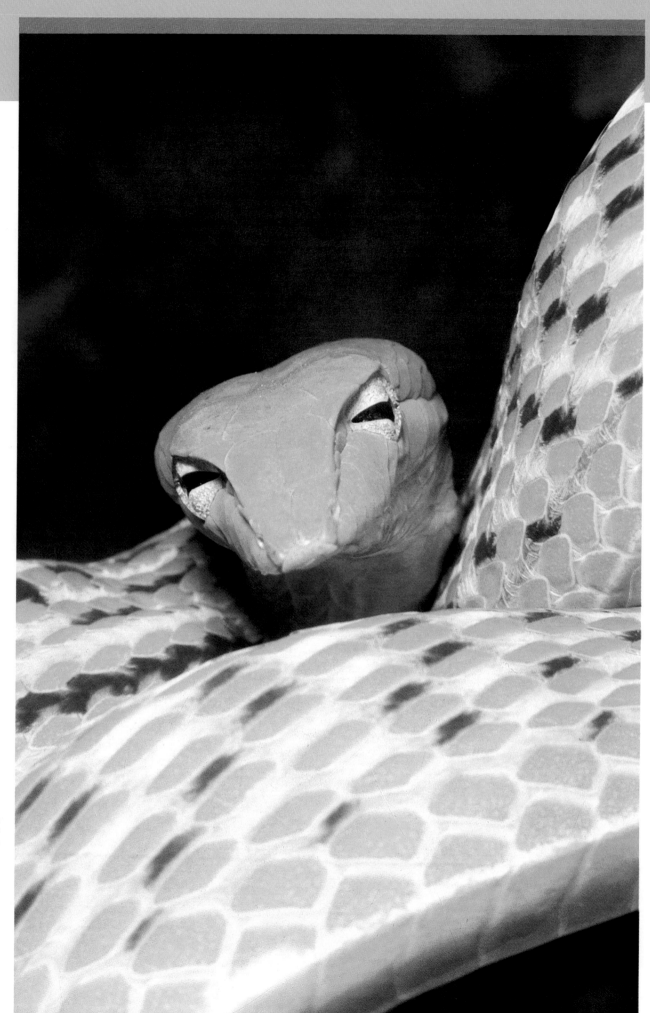

The vine snake has grooves in its head that extend from its eyes to its snout; they act like a sight on a gun barrel, improving its binocular vision.

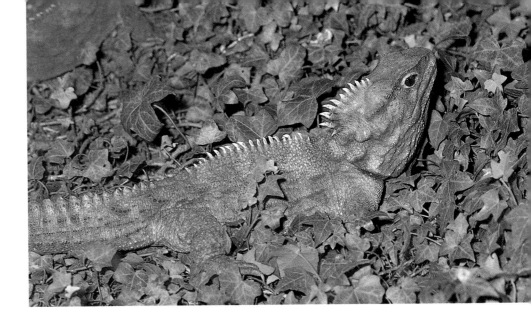

The tuatara lizard of New Zealand is the only lizard with a bona fide third eye, found on the top of its head. The eye has a covering lens, though image formation is very limited and the eye functions primarily as a hormonal clock.

in better focus. Tree snakes and bird snakes in particular also have excellent vision, as they must to catch birds. Tree and bird snakes have double foveas (circular concentrations of cone photoreceptors), one in the temporal area of the eye and the other centrally located. The temporal placement gives snakes like *Thelotornis kirtlandi,* and *Dryophis,* the beginnings of binocular vision. The emerald-green tree snake has the added advantage of two grooves cut down the sides of its nose, sort of like a gunsight. A muscle called the ventral transversalis pulls the lens toward the nose enabling the two ocular images to converge.

Sea snakes have a stenopeic pupil like the crocodile. The sea snake must be able to see clearly in water, where it finds its prey, but some of them also spend a considerable amount of time on land or swimming along the top of the water. Nature finally found a mechanism in the slit/stenopeic pupil that permits vision both in and out of water. It took centuries for nature to transform the original amphibian lens into one that functioned well on land; yet if the amphibian returned to water, it suffered a loss of acuity. The stenopeic pupil is nature's latest solution for animals who need to see well in both media.

The seal shares these same characteristics. Underwater, the eye uses a slit pupil; but above water it shuts down to the stenopeic pupil.

Corneal refraction or lens accommodation becomes unimportant because the opening in the pupil is so small that the eye resembles a pinhole camera, perhaps the most primitive type of lens. But again, the stenopeic lens can function well only in broad daylight.

Despite the most trying of circumstances, the snake cannot weep tears; it is the only reptile without lachrymal glands. But snakes do have harderian glands that secrete an oily substance to cleanse the eye's surface. Snakes also do not have eyelids. These have fused together to form a transparent spectacle that covers the cornea. The problem is that this covering scratches and impairs the snake's vision. Duke-Elder, whose series of books *The Eye in Evolution* is one of the main studies in comparative vision, reports that a scientific acquaintance succeeded in polishing the spectacles of a number of snakes and that they seemed very grateful, even including resentful types such as boas and pythons.

Though descended from lizards, snakes have eyes that differ considerably from lizards'; no bony spherical structure holds the eye in place, and there is no conus papillarus to nourish the cornea; this is accomplished instead by the aqueous humor.

By the way, the iris of the snake is very colorful, continuing the skin pattern right into the eye itself; how-ever, this is something one might want to appreciate from a distance.

The Tuatara Lizard

The tuatara lizard of New Zealand is the only remaining member of an ancient class of lizards called Rhynchocephalia. It has very limited vision and low acuity. And yet is has the most perfect remains of a third eye on top of its head. This is a true eye with a transparent covering and photoreceptors. Other creatures, such as the western lizard in the United States and the lamprey, have the remains of a third or pineal-parietal eye, but they are all rather primitive; similarly, there is a vestigial third eye in the tadpole, but this disappears in adulthood.

Presumably the third eye has no great importance in image formation but rather functions more as a light-gatherer that activates the body's hormonal clock, which in the case of the tuatara lizard operates rather slowly. This primitive relic of an ancient age is so lethargic that it has been known to fall asleep while eating. It matures sexually only at age 20 and is thought to have a lifespan of 100 to 300 years. Most of its life is spent hibernating, but the third eye never shuts, perhaps monitoring changes in light that tell this lizard when it's time to wake up.

10 *Birds*

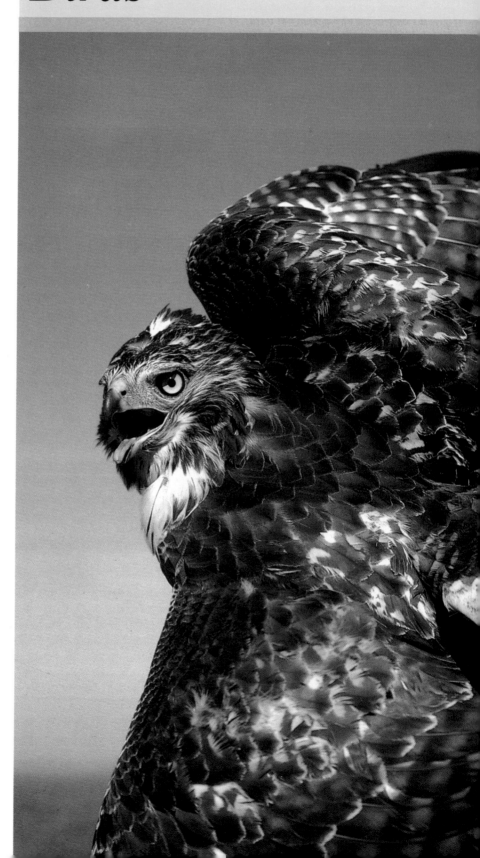

Ornithologists have described them as "flying eyes." Little escapes the gaze of a raptor, or predatory, bird such as the hawk, falcon or eagle. Supposedly, a vulture can spot a carcass from 3,000 to 4,000 meters in the air (at which height the bird can't even be seen by a human being on the ground). Medieval falconers carried a bird to see a bird; the frightened screams of the shrike alerted them to the return of the falcon long before the master could see it himself. Yet if the eye of the bird has attained a high state of development, it has been at the expense of its brain; think of our expression, "bird-brained."

All birds can be described as warm-blooded, back-boned vertebrates with two sets of limbs; one set has been modified with feathers to form wings while the other has become scaly legs, a throwback to the reptiles from which birds descended. Birds can be separated into two types: those that fly and those that walk or run. The largest eye of any land creature in the world belongs to a runner, the ostrich. The kiwi of New Zealand, another flightless bird, is the only winged creature that is myopic; most other birds are farsighted.

To better understand the subtle variations in vision among birds, we will consider them in five groups: passerine, or songbirds; predatory birds; seabirds; nocturnal birds; and domesticated birds. But first some visual characteristics shared by all birds.

The Eye of the Bird

The avian eye still has many similarities to the reptilian eye. Its shape is not spherical like the mammal's, though its shape varies among species. A ring of bony plates called spherical ossicles surround the eye, compensating for the flatness of the cornea and holding the eye rigid. The flattened shape of the avian eye makes it possible for it to maintain its entire visual field in focus at the same time, something that is impossible for the mammal, whose round eye can see clearly in only one small area of its visual field. Two layers of sclera, or outer coat, protect the eye, and the choroid layer is responsible for nourishing the retina.

A major improvement in the eye of the bird is the positioning of the lens. It has been pushed forward, closer to the cornea, which increases the size of the image on the retina. This improvement is retained in the eyes of mammals. But accommodation in the eye of the bird is superior to that of most, if not all, mammals. Accommodation might best be described as the range over which perfect focus can be maintained. (Seabirds have by far the greatest range, but predatory birds can see farther.) Two sets of ciliary muscles are at work to change focus: Brucke's muscles change the shape of the lens, which is common to many vertebrates, but some birds have a second set of ciliary muscles, called Crampton's muscles, that can also change the shape of the cornea. The hawk has both types of muscle, and this is just one of the many reasons for the amazing acuity of its vision. An adjunct to the ciliary muscles opens or closes the iris to admit more or less light, though for some reason the enlargement of the bird's pupils seems to reflect more its emotional state than the amount of available light.

Of all animals, birds have the largest number of photoreceptors in their retinas, with the hawk buteo as clear champion at 1,000,000 per sq mm. The tiny sparrow has 400,000 per sq mm, double the density in the human eye. But visual acuity is not dependent only on the number of exterior photoreceptors but also on how much of that information gets through to the brain via the bipolars and ganglion cells. Most birds have an aston-

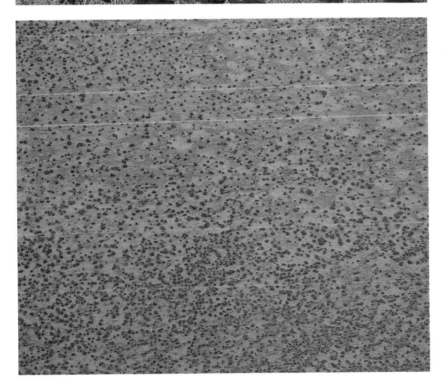

The hawk's vision is sometimes estimated to be eight times as sharp as our own. They have many more photoreceptors than we do and two foveas to our one. In fact, their foveas are so deep that they act as magnifiers. Here is a prairie seen from the point of view of a human and that of a hawk. Birds of prey can frequently see an object on the ground when we cannot even see the bird in the air.

ishingly high ratio of ganglion cells to photoreceptors; the peripheral retina of the white wagtail has 100,000 ganglion cells to 120,000 photoreceptors. This means that most of what the bird's eye sees is transmitted to the vision centers of its brain.

The avian eye has an unusual organ not found in any other eye and whose function is still something of a mystery. The pecten is a piece of folded tissue with many blood vessels that projects from the retina into the vitreous body. Pectens vary in shape, size and number of folds according to species. For example, the pectens of chickens have 18 folds, those of pigeons, 15 to 18, and so on. They are particularly developed in diurnal birds. Some scientists suggest that, since the pecten casts a shadow over the retina, it protects the eye from the dazzlement of too much light. Others maintain that their many blood vessels indicate that they feed the retina as the conus papillarus does in some reptiles. Still others have suggested that the pecten is an erectile organ that helps change the shape of the bird's eye for near and far vision. To date, there is no consensus.

Foveas are circular areas of the retina where large numbers of photoreceptors are gathered in one place, constituting the sharpest portion of the visual field. They are usually round and form a slight depression in the retina. Given their large numbers of photoreceptors, it should not be surprising that 95 percent of all birds have foveas and that only 54 percent have but one in each eye. A surprisingly large number of birds are bifoveate, including hummingbirds as well as hawks. (Besides eating nectar, the hummingbird captures insects on the wing on the tip of its tongue.) A central fovea gives high resolution to what is seen on either side of the head, while the temporal fovea improves binocular vision in front. Seabirds have another high concentration of photoreceptors in addition to two foveas; this is the horizontal visual streak that is generally found in creatures that need to scan a horizon.

In proportion to its body, the eye of the bird is larger than that of any other diurnal vertebrate. The rule of thumb for the camera-lens type of eye found in vertebrates is: The larger the eye, the greater its resolving power and thus its acuity. In fact, the eye of the bird has become so large that it cannot be moved in the socket, and the bird is forced to turn its head to follow a moving object. (Much of the bird's eye is concealed behind its skull and is not visible).

To what does the bird owe the incredible acuity of its vision? Certainly the complexity of flight, landing and catching prey on the wing require many immediate visual judgments. In fact, most of a bird's behavior is triggered by what the eye sees. Vision science refers to processes conducted within the eye as "coding," while those mediated by the central nervous system and neocortex are described as "thinking." Perhaps the visual judgments required of a bird leave little time for reflection. Anyone who has seen a bird swerve to avoid a moving car cannot help but appreciate this coding. The visual requirements of airborne creatures are far different from those who have their feet planted firmly on the ground.

The bird has upper and lower eyelids. The bottom eyelid is hidden and sweeps the eye like a wiper. It is present in man as a tear duct. The bird's eye also retains a light-shielding membrane found in reptiles, the nictitating membrane. Nocturnal birds use this membrane to protect their eyes from glare during daylight, while birds that spend long periods in the air (seabirds may fly on for days) cover their eyes with the membranes to protect them from foul weather and debris. The bird has harderian glands as well as lachrymal glands, with the former producing an oily substance that coats and protects the eye from dryness. Aqueous and vitreous humors, the jellylike substances found in all eyes, help maintain the shape of the eye. So much for the structure of the bird's eye. With minor varia-

tions—nocturnal birds have a fixed-focus lens—this is the basic anatomy. Oil droplets found in the individual cone photoreceptors may perform such an important function that they are discussed separately in the next section on avian color vision.

Color Vision in Birds

Perception of color among vertebrates reaches its height in the eye of the bird. The oil droplets found in individual cones are a much more flexible system of restricting short wavelengths than are the yellow filters that cover both the lens and macula lutea (a second filter in front of the retina) in man's eye: Whereas the human filters absorb all light below 400nm, oil droplets permit a highly selective screening of short-wavelength light rather than excluding all of it from the eye.

While the normal human eye has three basic cone types, the partnerships formed between oil droplets and varying pigment of different cones may create as many as five to seven different color classes in the bird's eye. Oil droplets also intensify some colors and exclude others. For example, birds with large numbers of red oil droplets see blues and violets as weak and desaturated. Some birds, such as the hawk, woodpecker and certain parrots, have few red oil droplets and probably see blues and violets much as we do. Red droplets are common in the eyes of pigeons and seabirds, who may fly for hours across water or in fog; these greatly improve their contrast vision.

▶

This vulture has its nictitating membrane drawn completely over its eyes. Nictitating membranes are used to keep out bright light during the day, to protect the eye from dust during flight and, in some diving birds, to change the refractive power of the eye when diving underwater.

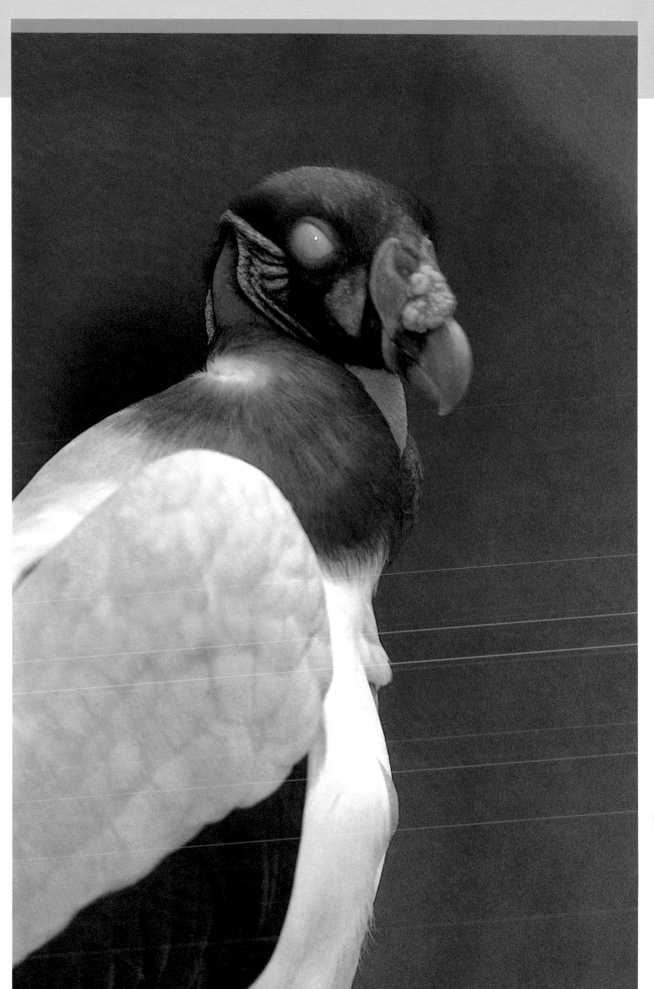

There are several schools of thought that believe that oil droplets have more than just a filtering function. These scientists suggest that the tiny droplets are actually microlenses improving the eye's sensitivity to light and motion and that, specifically, the oil droplets found in double cones increase the chances of photon capture. However, this is thought to be the case only with the double cones—two cones that grow together and are divided into a larger and a smaller, or accessory, cone. Such cones are also common in fish and amphibians.

The Perception of Polarized Light

A far more important function of oil droplets may be the detection of the plane of polarized light, again in concert with the double cone. For years vision scientists have wondered how pigeons and seabirds fly for hours, sometimes even days, in foggy skies. We know that birds use the sun for orientation and even have an excellent sense of time, since the sun shifts 15 degrees every hour. But how can they tell the sun's position when fog whites out the sky?

Until recently it was thought that the perception of polarized light was limited to invertebrates, albeit as diverse as bees and cephalopods; invertebrates with pigment located on layers of microbutules set at right angles to each other are able to gauge the direction of individual photons. But a modern theory suggests that the oil droplet in the principal cone of the bird scatters light that illuminates the accessory cone (which does not have an oil droplet), which absorbs it on a transverse angle and thus judges the direction from which the photon has come. While this is still only a theory, it is the best explanation we have of the extraordinary navigational abilities of so many species of birds.

Predatory Birds

There is something fierce about the look of the predatory, or raptor, birds. For years they have been depleted by indiscriminate hunting, though that period may be coming to an end. Their eyes are positioned on the front of their head, giving them excellent binocular vision, and they are bifoveate, with a central fovea used for lateral vision and a temporal fovea to improve their already excellent binocular vision.

The foveas of predatory birds are deeply indented into their retinas. The result is to magnify any part of the visual field reflected there. It may

Seabirds divide into those that dive for their food and those that simply skim fish from the top of the water. Some of the divers, like the goosander, will swim right after their prey underwater.

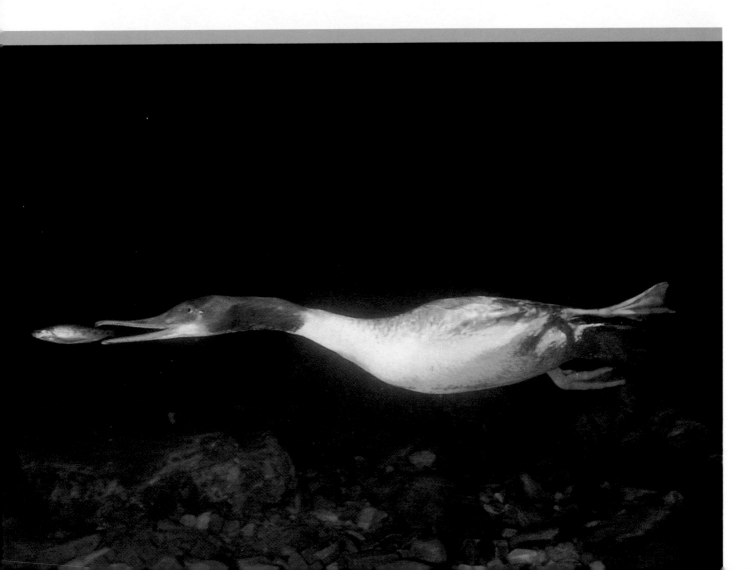

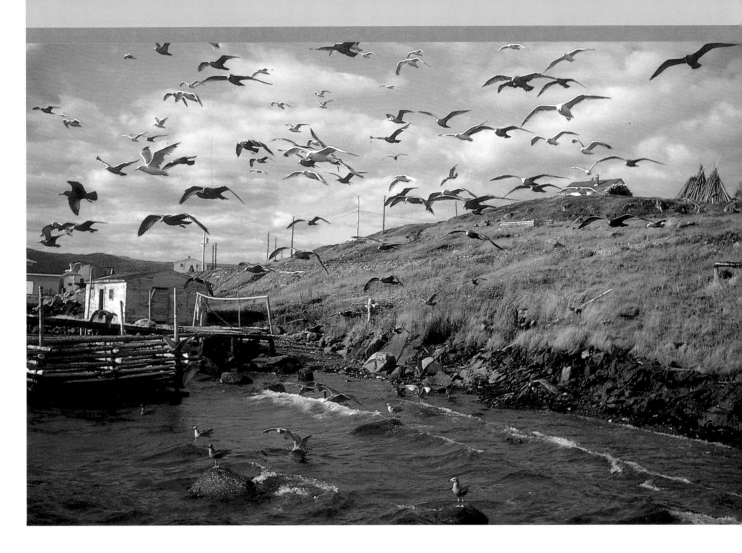

▲

Herring gulls, like pigeons and some other seabirds, have red oil droplets in their photoreceptors, which heighten contrast, improving their ability to navigate over long distances.

also distort what is seen, but if a bird is looking for food several miles high in the air, that may not be much of a problem. How the bird compensates once it is close to its prey is another question. Perhaps that is a matter of learned behavior; we already know that the archerfish learns to compensate for refraction when it spits at insects who fly above the surface of the water.

Falcons, hawks and eagles have few if any red oil droplets, though they do have some yellow and orange ones. It is therefore thought that they are unable to perceive polarized light and

probably see blues and violets much as we do. Judging from the drab color of these birds, color vision may be less important to them than it is to songbirds. The former's coloration may be described as earth tones: browns and grays relieved only by white; also, raptor birds evidently do not use color for sexual display as it is used in other birds.

What is extraordinary about predatory birds is the acuity of their vision. Some vision scientists claim that their peripheral vision is twice as good as ours while the frontal vision may be eight times as accurate. Certainly there are enough reasons for this acuity: huge numbers of photoreceptors in the retina; a high ratio of photoreceptor cells to bipolar and ganglion nerve cells; a bifoveate retina; a flatter cornea, which enables them to keep the total visual field in focus at the same time. Had birds developed

brains to match this formidable eye, there is no doubt that our early mammalian ancestors would have been in serious trouble.

Seabirds

Seabirds can maintain perfect focus over a greater distance than any other bird if not any other creature. The cormorant, which must contend with the change in refraction between air and water when it dives for fish, has a range of 50 diopters. (A diopter is a measurement of the refracting power of a lens; the larger the range of diopters of a lens, the greater the distance over which an eye can maintain perfect focus.) While the kingfisher does not have the same focal range as the cormorant, it is the only bird, if not the only creature, that

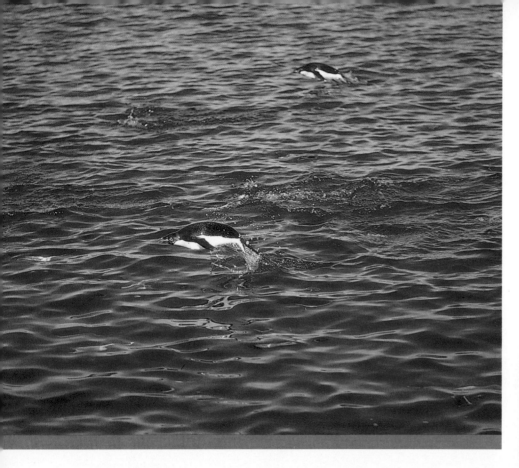

 The vision of penguins is better adapted to water than to land. Here two Adélie penguins leap through the water, looking more like the dolphin whose body resembles their own.

can see as well on land as in the water. This remarkable bird can dive for a fish and swim after it without losing visual acuity. Like so many other birds, the kingfisher is bifoveate and uses the central fovea for vision in the air but switches to its temporal fovea underwater. The lens of the kingfisher is egg-shaped, pointing to the temporal fovea, which means that its vision may even be superior in water. Other diving birds, such as auks, ducks and loons, place the transparent but highly refractive nictitating membrane over their eyes when they dive, increasing the resolution power of their lens in water.

Seabirds must be able to contend with weather and sea conditions that make vision difficult. It is easier for a fish to see out of water than for another creature, even a bird with incredible vision to see underwater.

First, objects seen from the water look smaller while those seen from the air appear bigger. Also, on a sunny day the glare reflected from the surface of the water is a problem. If it is windy and the water is choppy, there are myriad patterns of refraction. On a cloudy or foggy day, water and sky seem to merge; yet seabirds do find fish.

Seabirds can be separated into two types—those who feed from the surface and those who pursue fish underwater. Of those who pursue fish underwater, only 20 percent have red oil droplets, such as the shag, razorbill and shearwater, in addition to the kingfisher and cormorant already mentioned. Of those that feed from the surface, such as gulls and terns, 50 percent to 80 percent have red oil droplets. These birds must be able to see at great distances to locate plankton, whose presence produces a noticeable change in the color of the water. Where there is plankton, there will be tuna and other fish. The red oil droplets also increase the contrast sensitivity of the eye and enable birds to see through haze.

Apparently there is a correlation between the pale coloration of many seabirds and the presence of red oil droplets. White is the color prominent in these particular birds' sexual displays, and it happens that white birds are far more conspicuous than darker birds to others with red droplets. This may account for the dark coloration of baby birds, as a means of camouflage.

Seabirds that dive are much darker in color; they have few if any red droplets because water acts as a filter excluding the longer wavelengths that are passed with red oil droplets. The desaturation of blues caused by red droplets would be an advantage to birds who skim their food from the top of the water, since the dark fish would stand out; but birds that dive for food would be unable to see well once they penetrated the surface.

Gulls and terns have been studied in their nests off the coast of England, and a remarkable piece of behavior has been noted in connection with their feeding habits: The beaks of the mature birds are marked with a yellow and red spot which the nestling instinctually pecks when hungry. The parent responds by opening its beak and feeding the offspring. Experiments have shown that the baby will peck at other yellow and red spots and that this instinct is genetically coded rather than learned.

This eagle owl of Belgium has pulled its nictitating membrane over one eye while the other remains clear.

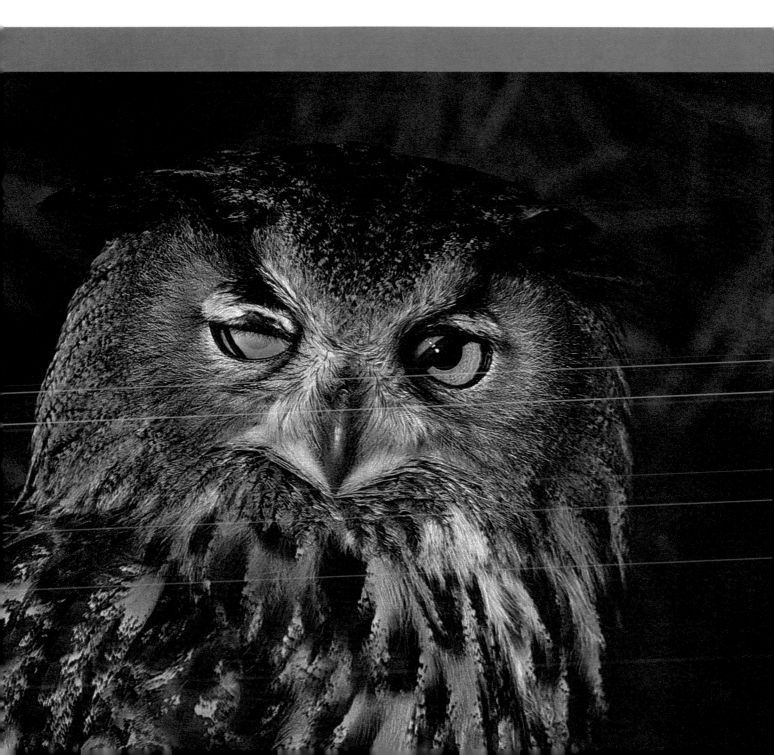

The penguin has a most unusual body for a bird; it resembles the dolphin more than other birds, and of course the penguin swims rather than flies, though its movements have been described as "flight underwater." The vision of penguins is adapted for water, and they are very nearsighted in air. The penguin's eyes are positioned on either side of its head, giving it a fairly wide visual field but very little binocular overlap, and the Adélie penguin has no binocularity at all.

How then does the very nearsighted Adélie trek hundreds of miles over what appears to us as featureless snow and locate the same spot where it nested the previous year? How can the adult pick out its offspring from 100 to 200 other baby penguins in the rookery? Perhaps they squint.

Nocturnal Birds

The eye of the quintessential bird of the night, the owl, has grown so large it has had to change shape and has become tubular. There is only so much room in the head even for a creature with little neocortex. (The eye of the owl resembles that of many deep-sea fish. There appear to be certain basic shapes for eyes that allow increased chances of photon capture whether they are miles below the sea or are limited to star- and moonlight.) To follow a moving creature, the owl simply turns its head and looks over its shoulder, a mobility it shares with another nocturnal creature, the tarsier of Asia.

The owl is one of the few birds with any significant binocularity. As the eyes have grown, they have pushed toward the front of its face until they now have a frontal overlap of 60 to 70 degrees. Its visual field is very limited, only 110 degrees in contrast to the parrot, for example, which has a combined visual field of 300 degrees. The reason for this limitation lies in the structure of its tubular eyes. Visual fields are dependent on the angular extension of the retina, which is very limited in the tubular eye. In fact, deep-sea fish have an accessory retina on the side, sort of a "side-view mirror," which has not evolved in the owl. In fact, the limited nature of the owl's visual field may be one reason why nature has improved the mobility of its neck. Still, binocularity is very important to a nocturnal animal since it increases the resolution of the area of visual overlap.

While great attention has recently been paid to the owl's outstanding hearing, its primary sense is vision. The owl has excellent vision at night and probably sees better than we do even during the day, except where color contrast is needed. The rods in its retina are very fine and closely packed, which makes for an excellent optical image on the retina comparable to a finely grained black-and-white photograph. The owl has no color vision and presumably no cones in its retina at all. Creatures with rod vision have an advantage over those with cone-rich retinas in that the latter are blind at night while nocturnal creatures have some vision (the owl, excellent vision) all day.

Nocturnal birds have few if any colored oil droplets in their retinas; the owl has clear oil droplets. Filters block out light, and the last thing any nocturnal creature needs is to lose any light at all. Red, yellow and orange droplets tend to increase contrast, something that is unnecessary to the nocturnal eye. But the owl does have a reflecting tapetum that directs more light to the retina.

There are comparatively few other nocturnal birds, though there are some that are considered crepuscular, i.e., that are active at dawn or in early evening: nightjars, swallows and swifts. The *Apus apus* has particularly good vision and captures insects on the wing as it skims over the surface of the water. We are more accustomed to the sound of birds as we wake at dawn, but the nightingale, as one might conclude from its name, is also crepuscular.

It should be noted that the focal range of nocturnal and crepuscular birds is far more limited than that of

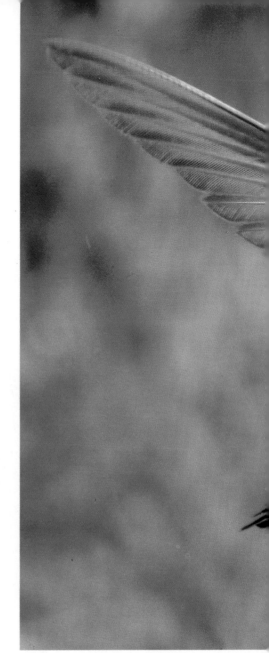

▲

Though the hummingbird, an important pollinator of many plants, shows a strong attraction to the color red, this may only be learned behavior. Recent experiments show that their eyes have ultraviolet receptors.

predatory or seabirds. The former's vision is generally good over a range of three diopters; the exception is four—quite a difference from the 50 diopters of the cormorant.

Nocturnal birds also have fixed-focal-length lenses, since the ciliary muscles to accommodate for near and far vision are lacking. Consequently, when the owl eats, it must pull back its head to see its food clearly.

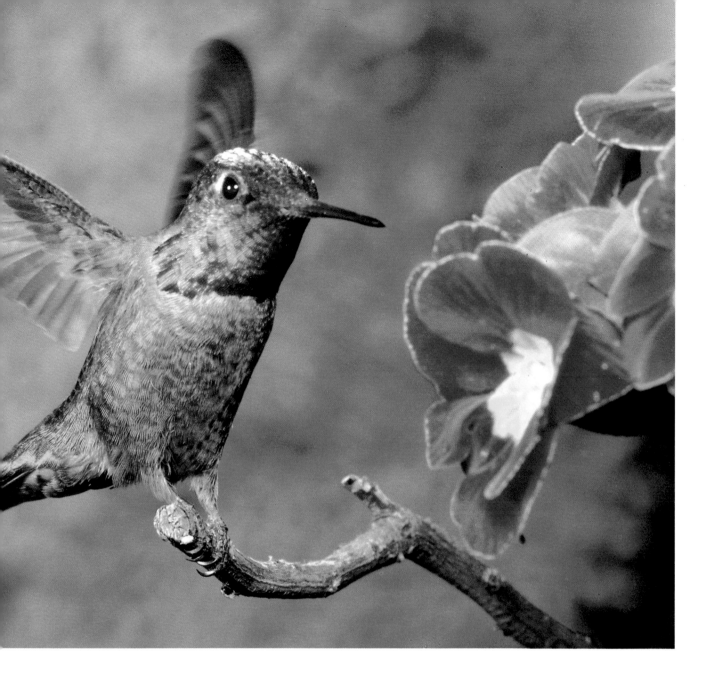

Celestial Navigation

Observation and experimentation in planetariums have shown that birds navigate by the stars and know their positions. Dr. Sauer of Freiburg University raised night-migrating warblers in confinement, then took them to a planetarium with projected replicas of the major stars. The baby birds adjusted their position to the direction in which the parents were already flying. When he changed the positions of the stars, the birds readjusted themselves. Other experiments with various species of night-flying birds have replicated the results of these experiments, some of which were conducted in exterior cages under the stars.

It requires an extremely large eye to detect small points of light at great distances, and the eye of the bird is certainly big enough to perceive starlight. What is of greater interest in the experiments of Dr. Sauer is that knowledge of the stars' positions appears to be innate, like the innate attraction of young gulls to yellow and red spots.

Passerine, or Songbirds

It is apparent from their own coloration that color vision plays an important role in the life of the songbird. Color is used for sexual display; an unusual example is the bowerbird, which fills its nest with colorful objects but knows that the female prefers blue. Also, many plants use birds as pollinators; there are at least 150 species of plants that use birds as pollinators in Patagonia, Brazil, South Africa and Australia, and sixty types of hummingbirds per-

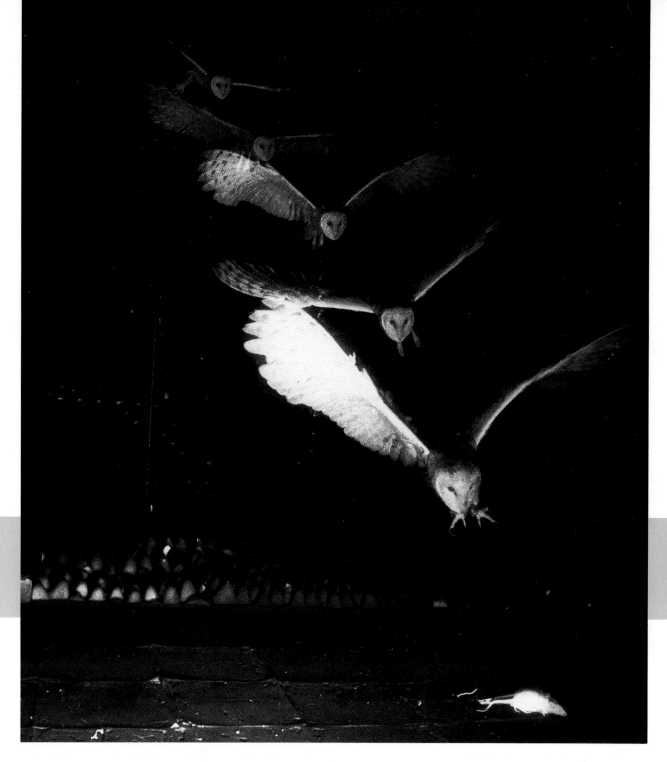

form the same function in the United States. Ripe fruit and conspicuously colored seeds signal these birds that the plant is ready for the eating (and pollination).

As we have learned in the study of insects, color is more recognizable to creatures moving swiftly through the air than is form, but color combined with form is even more easily discernible. Spring is short, and one must find a mate swiftly if one's genes

are to be passed on; oil droplets in the songbirds pass the colors found in members of its own species better than it does other colors. Oil droplets are generally red, orange, yellow, green or blue. Red droplets predominate in the hummingbird, which seems particularly drawn to red flowers; in fact, some can see also the ultraviolet down to a range of 370nm. Remember that oil droplets are a very selective form of filtration; they give the humming-

▲

In this photograph, taken under infrared light with infrared film, we see a barn owl in the process of capturing a mouse. Owls are thought to see into the near infrared. As a result, they can see in the dark, where we would have no vision. Also, there is no doubt that hearing also plays an important role in the owl's ability to function at night, but vision is its primary sense. The other photo shows three juvenile barn owls.

bird a range of color vision far exceeding our own.

The eyes of songbirds are farther apart than birds of prey's and the former have minimal binocularity; the parrot's is just about nine degrees. However, their range of vision is greater than that of the nocturnal bird, extending from 8 to 12 diopters.

Domesticated Birds

Domesticated chickens and other fowl kept in pens tend to nearsightedness, unlike most other birds with the exception of the kiwi. Domestic birds' retinas contain red, yellow and orange oil droplets, which means that blues and violets appear less saturated than the longer-wavelength colors. Domestic fowl seem to be born with an innate sense of the shape of feed grains and will ignore food lit so that its shadow is removed. The jerking motion that fowl make from side to side is to better see their food; they are changing angles to correct for parallax. Like the owl, they have great difficulty focusing on objects that are very close.

We know from Sumerian tablets that the pigeon has long served man as a messenger. Its homing abilities are legendary. On a clear day, it uses the position of the sun as a guide, but it is equally adept on a foggy day when you or I would easily get lost. If the already-mentioned theory concerning polarized light is correct, the pigeon, with its large number of double cones and red oil droplets, probably locates the sun through the direction of photons.

The pigeon has so many red droplets in the forward and bottom sections of its retina that they are described as a red field. The rest of the retina is dominated by yellow droplets. Red droplets cut off wavelengths below 580nm, which means that the pigeon has practically no appreciation of violets and blues. Its best color perception occurs around 600nm, where it can distinguish colors separated by as little as 3nm.

Pigeons are herbivorous and must be able to identify a variety of plants. The pigeons' filters absorb greens, but since plants also reflect biochromes (substances found in nature that reflect specific wavelengths of light) other than chlorophyll, such as anthocyanins and carotenoids, which reflect reds, yellows and oranges (pigments responsible for the subtle variations of colors in leaves), the birds can nevertheless differentiate various types of flora.

Vision science has shown great interest in the eye of the pigeon, and numerous experiments have been conducted over the years with interesting results. For example, we know that a pigeon can distinguish among many different photographs and that it is faster than any human at identifying mirror writing or mirror images. Again, there is obviously something to be said for visual coding.

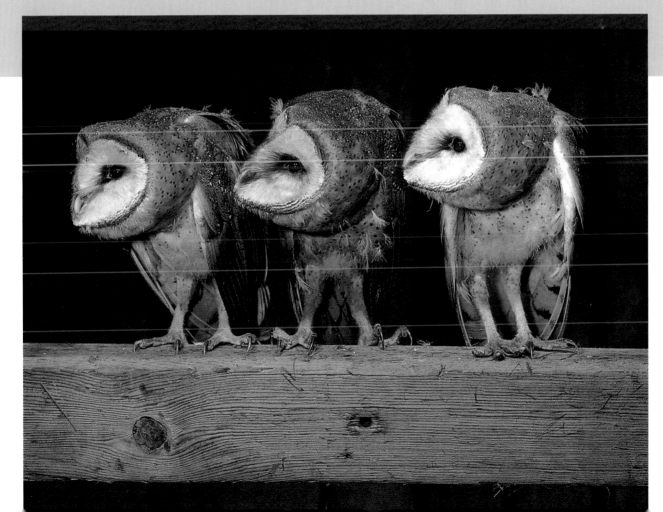

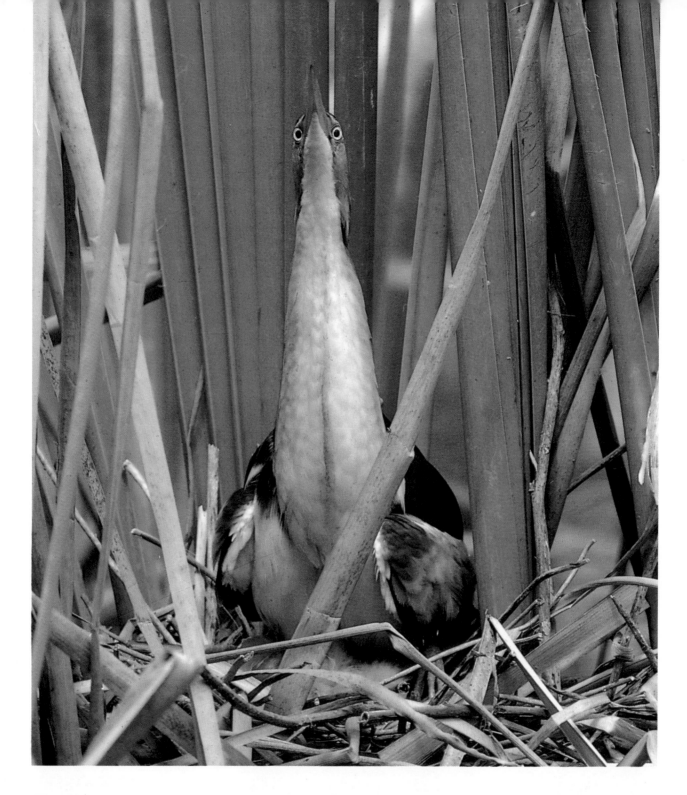

The Unusual Eyes of the Bittern and the Snipe

Some characters do not fit easily into any category, and such is the case with the bittern and the snipe. The eyes of the snipe are set so far back in its head that it has *rear* binocular vision while it is eating. Visual overlap in front is one thing, but this bird has depth perception behind its head. Then there's the bittern. It's eyes are set far apart on either side of its beak, and under normal conditions this feathered creature would have no binocularity at all. But it has discovered that by raising its beak high in the air and looking underneath it, it gets a better look. Thus, the female in the adjacent photo could

▲

The bittern's eyes are positioned so far on either side of its head that it must raise its beak and look under it to get any sort of binocular overlap.

watch her babies in the nest below her as she studied the photographer in front of her.

11

Nocturnal Animals

Even on the brightest moonlit night, the amount of light available for vision is millions of times less than during daylight. The stars above us add little in the way of light for vision, yet celestial navigation, the gift of the starry night, has not been used only by man. We know from experiments in planetariums that some birds navigate by the constellations. But most nocturnal animals do not enjoy good image formation. Rather, nature has sacrificed visual acuity in order that these creatures have any vision at all.

The Dark-Adapted Eye

Most creatures active at night are either decendants of animals who fled to the relative safety of the dark or those who pursued them there. Since there is less light available at night, nature was very accommodating: It made the nocturnal eye larger, in some cases so big that it could no longer move in its socket. To follow a moving object the animal was forced to twist its neck; hence tarsiers and owls can turn their heads almost completely around and stare behind them. In addition, the pupil was widened. A camera lens is considered fast, that is, able to shoot with little available light, with an F-stop of 1.4. Our own eye has its best

▶

The eyes of the tarsier have become so enormous that they cannot be moved in their sockets. But to compensate, this nocturnal creature, like the owl, can swivel its neck almost 360 degrees, thus enabling it to see all around.

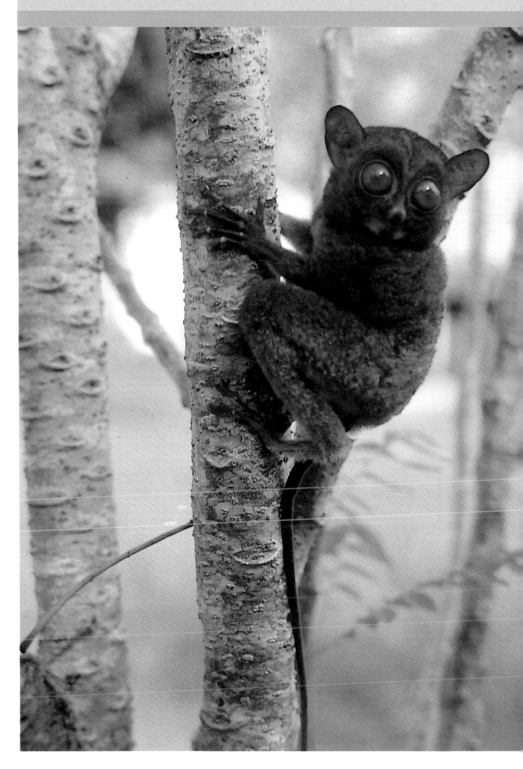

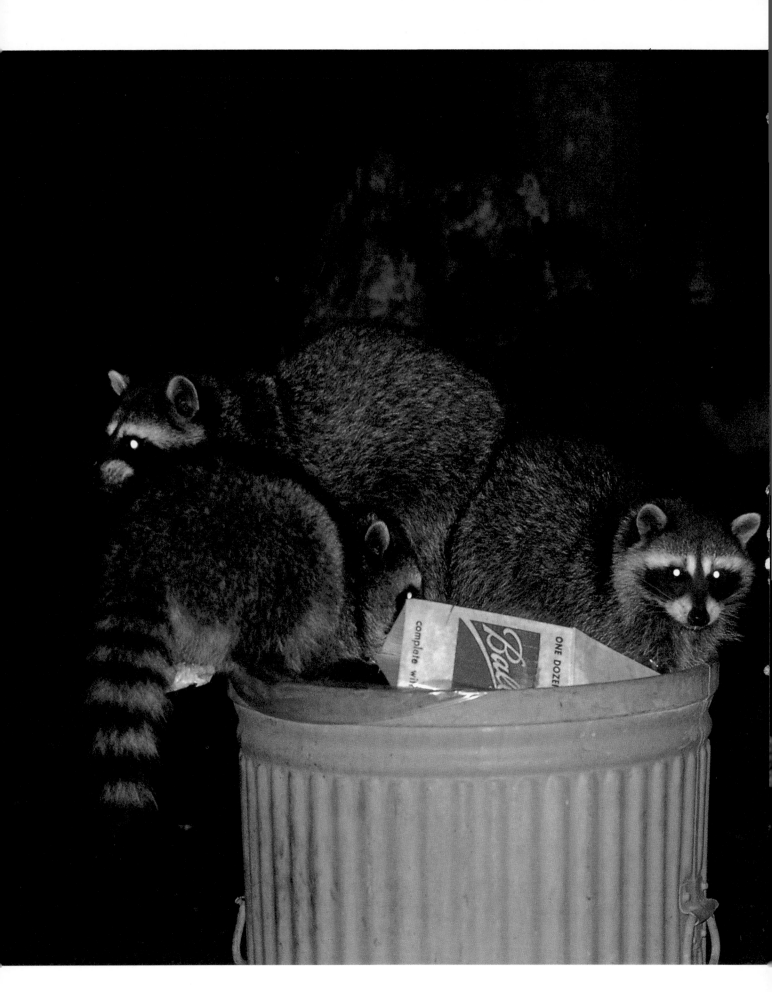

resolution at approximately f2.4, but the cat has an f-stop of .09; a nocturnal moth, f0.5; and the owl, f1.3.

However, these wide apertures put the nocturnal creature at risk if awakened during the day: Its rod photoreceptors can be damaged by too much light. The douricouli monkey of South America, one of the few nocturnal primates, will actually go blind if its eyes are kept open in daylight. Or a creature can be temporarily blinded by glare, a real disadvantage in a confrontation with a predator. Round pupils simply require too much muscular effort to squeeze into a small enough opening in daylight, so nature developed the slit pupil. Most of us have seen the extreme change in a cat's pupils when they are exposed to bright light. Another protection from glare is the nictitating membrane, an opaque fold of skin that covers the eye, almost like an eyelid. This natural device is found mostly in nocturnal birds, reptiles and amphibians, and present in only some mammals.

The corneas and lenses of nocturnal animals are huge in comparison to those of diurnal animals. Every effort is made to capture those few photons available for vision. Also, the retinas of nocturnal animals consist of all, or nearly all, rods. Why rods? Cones, the color photoreceptors, require too many photons to fire. At night they become quite useless. But the rods pool, or sum, their information to form an image. Large numbers of rods—in the case of deep-sea fish this can be thousands or even hundreds of thousands—connect to the next layer of cells in the eye, the bipolars. Because they share the same neural connection, the information sent forward by each rod has less of a chance of being received without modification. As a result, the picture they form has nowhere near the clar-

◀

The world of the night is black and white, and the markings of raccoons are typical of all nocturnal creatures. In this picture, we see the tapetal glow of their eyes in the camera flash.

ity of detail formed by a cone image; but to the nocturnal creature some sort of image is better than no image at all.

An interesting way to experience your own rod vision is to take a walk one moonlit night where there are no manmade lights. You will note that your best vision is out of the periphery of your eyes, where rods predominate, rather than from the center of the eye, the location of the cone-rich fovea.

Dark-adapted invertebrates generally have a better chance of absorbing photons than do dark-adapted vertebrates. For example, the lobster, a nocturnal invertebrate, has rhabdoms open in the direction of the lenslets of the ommatidia, while the rods of the vertebrate eye point instead in the direction of the brain. (In fact, one of the proofs that invertebrate and vertebrate evolution occurred separately is found in the structure of the eye: Rods and cones point toward the brain because the vertebrate eye is a direct outgrowth of the brain, while the invertebrate eye evolved instead from neural ectoderm—skin.) The plus for the invertebrate eye is a better chance of absorbing light, but the minus is its lack of a well-developed brain.

The Tapetum

Nature's nocturnal mirror, the tapetum, is even more necessary to the vertebrate eye. The type found in some marsupials and most mammals, such as whales, dolphins, predatory cats and ungulates (hooved, herbivarous creatures such as horses), is the tapetum fibrosum—a layer of mirrorlike reflecting cells imbedded in the choroid layer right behind the retina. While not as effective as the tapetum of fish and crocodiles, which is made of guanine crystals (a highly reflective material that is also the basis of a fish's scales), it nevertheless fulfills the function of

The tapetum causes the eye of nocturnal creatures to glow in the dark, and the color of the glow depends on

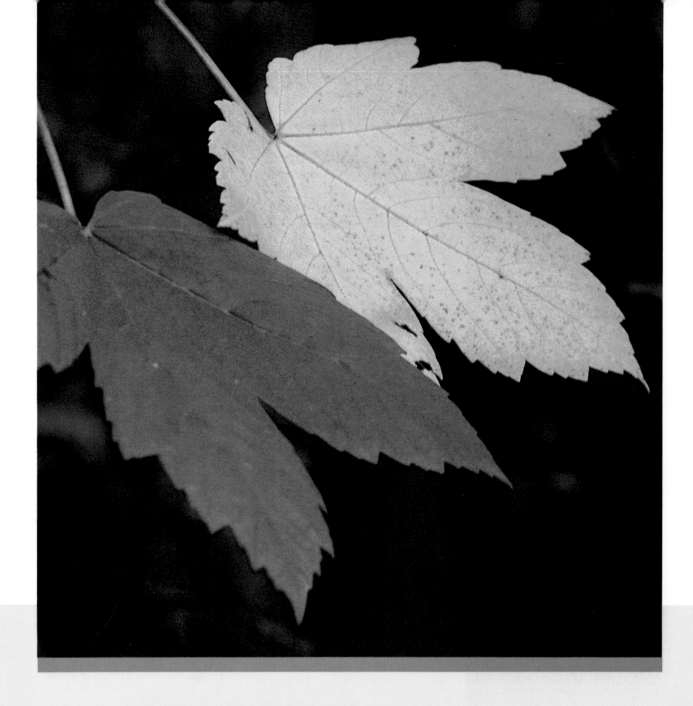

the coloration of the visual pigment in photoreceptors. Deep-sea fish have a golden visual pigment. The glow from the eyes of predatory cats, including our own domesticated versions, is golden; the rabbit's and the hare's is red; members of the lemur family have a golden yellow; an antelope's is white; and the hippo's is red.

Yet with all these advantages—enlarged eyes, expanded pupils, more rod photoreceptors, some of them very large in size—how well do nocturnal creatures see? Certainly far better than we do at night. But the nocturnal eye has paid a price for the increased sensitivity of its vision: It does not have great resolving power and cannot distinguish fine detail.

At night it takes more time to gather enough light to form an image. Therefore, if something moves very quickly against a static back-

▲ ▲

To the diurnal eye such as our own, the brightest of all colors is yellow, but to the nocturnal animal, green is the brightest color (right).

ground, it will not be seen (just as a moving object creates only a blur in a photograph taken at slow speed). During the day our own eyes can construct an image in .035 to .06 of a second, while at night it takes at least a tenth of a second.

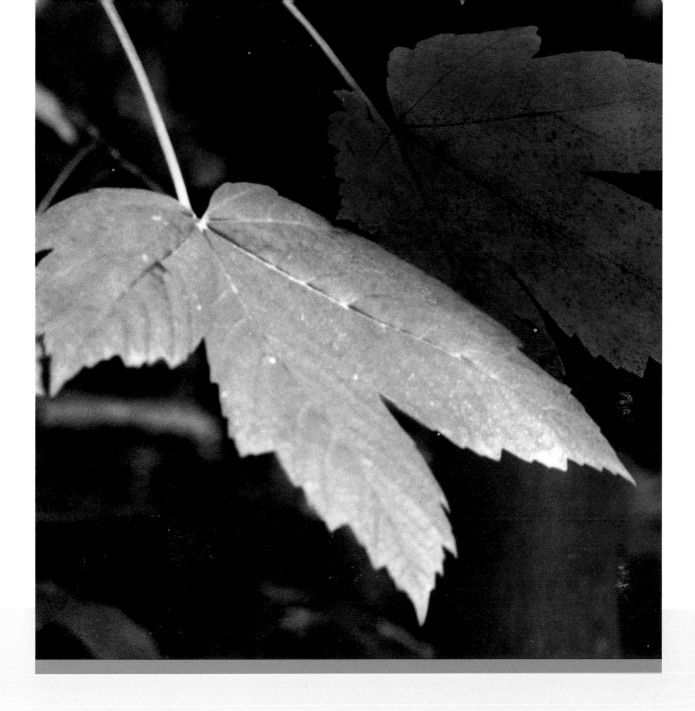

Color and the Dark-Adapted Eye

The world of the night is black and white. No color separates objects or other living creatures from their backgrounds. Plants pollinated by moths and bats are generally white and therefore more visible in the dark. Most nocturnal creatures are black, and if they have any markings they are generally gray or white. But even if these creatures see only in shades of gray and white, they can still differentiate colors from each other by their degree of brightness or luminosity.

Here we come to one of the most striking differences between the dark-adapted eye and the eye of the diurnal creature—the change in the relative brightness of colored objects. If we look at a yellow lemon and a green lime, the lemon appears the brighter of the two because yellow is the brightest color to the diurnal eye. But the vision of the dark-adapted eye has shifted to shorter wavelengths, and it sees green as the brightest color. While it may be difficult for us to imagine, when a fruit bat looks at a lemon tree, the green leaves are brighter than the lemons, and when a badger looks at a buttercup, the flower appears darker than the stem.

The Purkinje Shift

Creatures with duplex retinas, those that contain both rods and cones, undergo a transformation in the relative brightness of colors during the day and night. This transformation is called the Purkinje Shift, after its discoverer. During the day it is predominantly the cones that activate and dominate the neural channels to the brain. At night, the cones cease to function, and the rods are responsible for vision. During the day, yellow is the brightest color and reds are very visible, but at night, as in the dark-adapted eye, vision is shifted to the shorter wavelengths; green is the brightest color, and reds cannot be seen against a dark background. Rods contain only rhodopsin, whose absorption maximum is around 500nm, which means that wavelengths of light in the yellow, orange and red area of the spectrum are poorly perceived. It also accounts for the sudden blinding one experiences on entering or leaving a dark tunnel on a bright day; the rods or cones require a short period to activate.

The night is a busy place filled with a surprising number of creatures. Most spiders are nocturnal, as are many amphibians and reptiles, most marsupials and some mammals: all 981 species of bats, 60 percent of all species of carnivores, 40 percent of the 1,729 species of rodents, 20 percent of all species of primates and 80 percent of all species of marsupials (according to Jack Prince in *Animals of the Night*). In this chapter we will concern ourselves only with marsupials and mammals. For night vision in amphibians, reptiles and spiders, see the separate chapters on those creatures.

Nocturnal Marsupials

There are predatory marsupials like the fearsome Tasmanian devil, with its eyes positioned squarely in front of its head, and herbivorous marsupials, which, like other creatures of prey, have their eyes positioned on either side of their head to give them wider visual fields. It appears to be a truism that the predator's vision is generally better than that of its prey. Herbivorous creatures who depend on bulky plant food for their diet have a formidable problem: They are noisy eaters, and even if they can't be seen, they are certainly heard. Most marsupials are found in Australia; in the Americas we have the opossum, which is the only marsupial on the continent that managed to survive the advent of the placental mammal. When attacked, they pretend to be dead, "play possum"; apparently this is a successful ruse, for not only have they survived, they are on the increase. Possums are a more primitive type of marsupial, the polydont (many teeth), while kangaroos and wallabys are examples of a more advanced marsupial, the diprodont (two teeth), though they are not nocturnal.

However, more than just teeth separates these two types of marsupials. Polydonts have no connecting link between the two hemispheres of the brain, the means by which visual information is shared. As in all sub-mammalian species, their optic nerve from the left eye crosses over to the right hemisphere of the brain while the optic nerve from the right eye crosses over to the left hemisphere. Since there is no connecting link, there can be no coordinated eye movements and no simultaneous expansion or contraction of the pupils. Even if the eyes are placed frontally, the disparity of the two retinal images cannot be compared by the brain; therefore these creatures must use monocular visual cues for depth perception.

The diprodont does have a connecting link between the hemispheres, the anterior commissure. This enables them to share some visual information, but it is a very primitive linkage belonging to the oldest part of the brain. If one wonders why the placental mammals were able to displace the marsupials, this may be one of the reasons. The corpus callosum that connects the hemispheres of the mammalian brain is not only a superior linkage, but its activity enables the hemisphere of each side of the brain to locate visual information stored by the other side while employing some suppressive device so that both sides of the brain do not have to record the same memory, thus increasing the space available for visual memories. Not only is the anterior commissure an inferior linkage but both hemispheres of the brain must store the same information, using up available cortex more quickly.

In English as well as other languages there is more than one word for *seeing*. We *look* as well as *see*. What we are describing with these words is the effect of visual memory that somehow imprints itself in the brain. Lettvin (who along with McCulloh *et al.* is one of the authors of a scientific monograph called *What the Frog's Eye Tells the Frog's Brain*.) tells us that even frogs have a visual system that contains what he calls "sameness" neurons and "newness" neurons. Toads who have had the misfortune to eat bees learn to recognize and avoid them, but the optic fibers of amphibians connect to a region of the brain called the retino-tectal area, which is still a reflex center. In the mammalian brain, the entire retino-tectum (sometimes called the reptilian brain), has become only one small part, the superior colliculus, and the cortex, with its memory bank of associative neurons, in particular the visual cortex or area striata, has developed. The marsupial eye is really very much like the eye of many mammals (though it has no lens accommodation). But it is the brain's lack of a corpus callosum that is a major detriment to its visual system.

Bats

About an hour after sunset these strange-looking creatures leave their roosts in caves or buildings or wherever they have been able to spend a congenial day far from

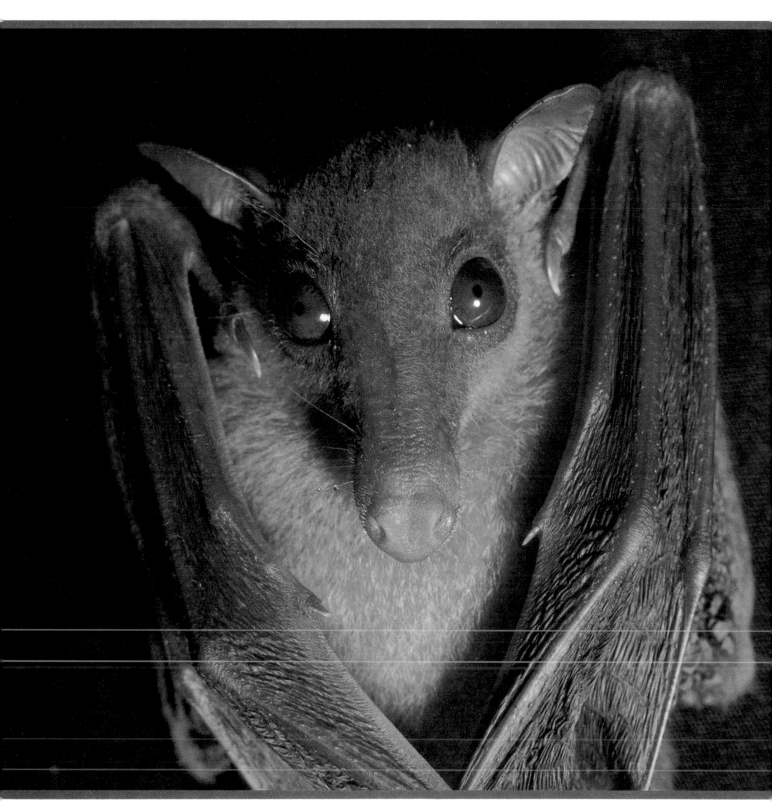

Bats are the only flying mammal, and most of them rely on echolocation to make their way. But there are fruit bats who rely solely on their eyes; and scientists have also discovered that covering the eyes of any bat causes it to fly erratically. Obviously, visual clues are more important to bats than is often thought to be the case.

heat or light. They flap through the darkening sky frequently mistaken for birds; for as birds dominate the daytime sky, it is the bat that dominates the night. It is the only flying mammal.

A common misconception is that bats do not see well. In fact, some, the Megachiroptera, or fruit, bat, see as well as any other mammal of their size. Their New World cousins, the Microchiroptera, or insectivorous, bats rely more on the use of echolocation, a highly sophisticated sonar system, to find food or avoid collision. These bats emits a series of clicking sounds that bounce against other objects and are played back to the bat at high frequencies not discernible to the human ear. (There are a number of moths who have learned to jam these frequencies by making similar clicking sounds.) Then the bat is forced to use its eyes.

Only one species of fruit bat is capable of echolocation, so most fruit bats rely on vision. Among these are the flying foxes of Southeast Asia. There is also a fishing bat whose vision is so sensitive it can detect the ripples of fish in water. So much for the myth of the blind bat. In fact, scientists have actually blindfolded bats who rely on echolocation and found that they fly erratically and can take much longer to find their way home. Obviously they use visual cues as well as echolocation to identify landmarks.

There is still some argument on the existence of lens accommodation in the bat's eye. Recently some vision scientists have asserted that fruit bats can change the shape of their lens, but the classic theory advanced by Walls in *The Vertebrate Eye* is that near and far vision in the bat is actually accomplished by the retina itself. When looked at under a microscope, the bat retina gives the appearance of ridges and valleys. Its

retina is described as corrugated, or papillated, with some of the photoreceptors farther from the lens than others. (Generally, nature goes to great lengths to make light fall uniformly on the retina.) Because of the varying position of the photoreceptors, some part of the visual image will be in focus for near objects and another part for far. Through experience, the bat can learn to vary its body distance from an object when it wants to see something clearly. This all sounds

very complicated. But what is truly extraordinary is the ability of the mother bat to locate her children in a darkened cave amid thousands of other baby bats.

Other Nocturnal Mammals

The most familiar nocturnal mammals are creatures like raccoons, badgers and skunks.

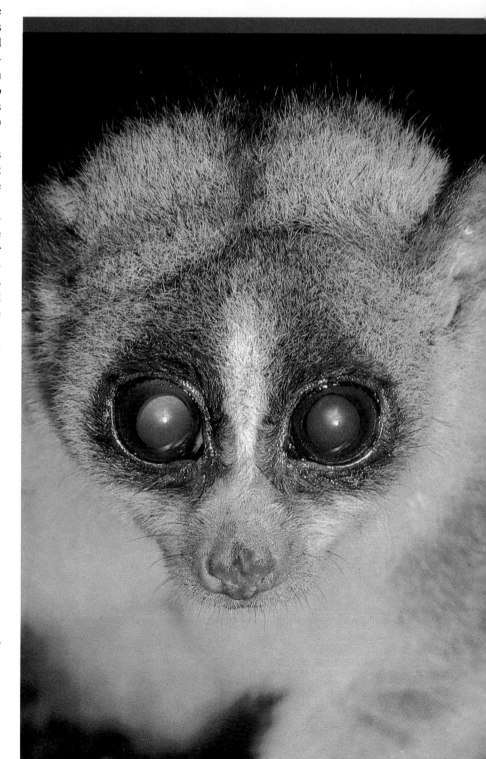

Like most prosimians, the lorises are nocturnal. Their vision is not as good as that of the tarsier, nor can they move as quickly, so they are sometimes referred to as the languid lorises.

The skunk and badger are black and white, while the raccoon is gray and black. Both animals blend easily into the night, except when the skunk uses the white in its tail for sexual display or as what one might call an early warning system before emitting the foul-smelling spray for which it is noted.

The vision of these creatures varies somewhat. The badger is a burrower, and its eyesight is very poor. It has no lens accommodation and little range of vision. The skunk's vision is better and its range farther. Its visual acuity is greater as well. The raccoon, like all creatures that use their paws for grasping, has some lens accommodation and a more complex brain and is capable of manipulating its environment, somewhat like the diurnal squirrel.

Despite these creatures' poor acuity, they each have the beginnings of depth perception found only in mammals, which will be discussed in greater detail in the next chapter, on diurnal mammals.

The douroucouli, a monkey of South America, is the only known nocturnal primate, and its eyes are so sensitive that if they are exposed to daylight for any length of time the animal can go blind.

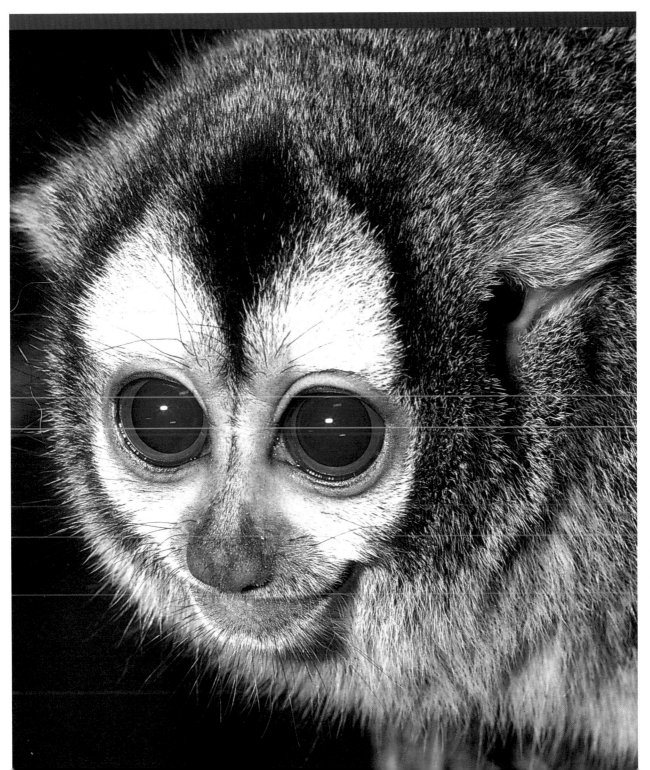

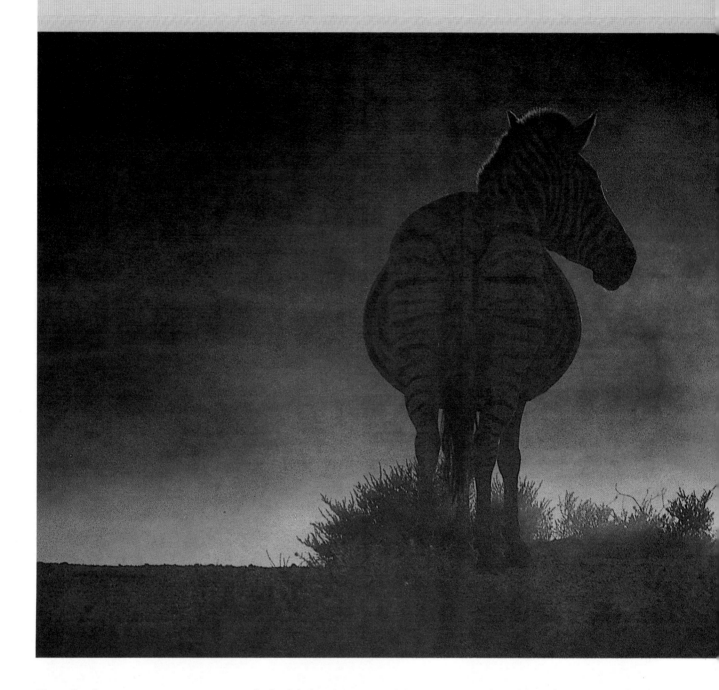

Prosimians

The prosimians are the earliest primates and are, with the exception of the diurnal lemur of Madagascar, nocturnal. The other diurnal prosimians were displaced by the onslaught of more aggressive diurnal apes, while the lemur was protected by the wall of water that surrounds its island home in the Indian Ocean.

Prosimians are found mainly in Africa and Asia. In Africa there are the bush baby, the potto and the angwantibo; in Ceylon the slow loris and the slender loris, both frequently referred to as the languid lorisines because of their slow pace. The tarsier of Southeast Asia has the largest eyes in proportion to its body of any living creature, 150 times bigger in proportion to its body than human eyes are to our body. They literally bulge out of its head. In fact, they are so large that, like the owl, the tarsier cannot move them in their sockets but is forced to twist its head to follow a moving object; it can turn 180 degrees and look over its shoulder. When its eyes are completely open in the dark, the iris is no more than a narrow band around the rim of the eye. Though most prosimians are insectivores, the tarsier likes meat and has the vision, speed and reflexes to catch small birds, rodents and lizards as well as insects; all of this in the pitch dark.

The African bush baby has fast reflexes and excellent night vision, though nowhere near the level of the tarsier. It moves quickly through the

At night, when the animals are most vulnerable, the zebras' stripes help to break up their silhouettes and camouflage them from prey.

mates and mammals. Like prosimians, it still relies as much on its sense of smell, but cones have been discovered in the retina, which is very unusual for a nocturnal creature, and it also has the beginnings of stereoscopic vision, which is found only in mammals and reaches its height in the primates. For a long while three-dimensional vision was considered part of image formation, till it was proven that its neural connections providing the brain with information about depth actually preceded image formation. But this should not be surprising. Nocturnal mammals have poor image formation in the first place, but depth perception would be a real advantage to a creature swinging through the jungle, especially at night. In contrast, monocular visual clues such as distance, interposition, texture and gradient would not work as well in the dark.

The earliest mammals did not choose life in the dark because their eyes saw better at night; they escaped to the nocturnal world because they had the capacity to make their own body heat, while the giant carnivorous reptiles who fed on them became torpid without the warmth of the sun. There, in a world lit only by the moon and stars, a world of outlines and silhouettes, shapes without detail, brightness without color, these creatures sought survival. Nature adapted their eyes accordingly. Moreover, some of the improvements were to prove even more valuable when the dinosaurs disappeared and mammals could once again emerge into the sunlight. Those who descended from life in the trees came better equipped for the transition than those who had remained on the ground.

jungle by jumps and leaps. In captivity it is known to ignore immobile crickets, though this may indicate only lack of interest: It took vision scientists a long time to realize that toads had color vision, because the animals got bored when the experiments were not varied.

The potto and angwantibo are both slow-moving climbers, though the potto has the better vision. These creatures subsist on bad-smelling insects ignored by the faster bush babies. It would be interesting to find out if any experiments have compared the lens accommodation of the faster-moving bush babies and slower lorisines to see if the ability to move and grab swiftly is matched by faster and greater lens accommodation. To my knowledge, such experiments have not been done.

Vision scientists, like other scientists, are always looking for links between species. *Tupaia glis,* a small nocturnal tree shrew with a shrunken snout and enormous eyes, is considered a possible link between pri-

12 *Mammals*

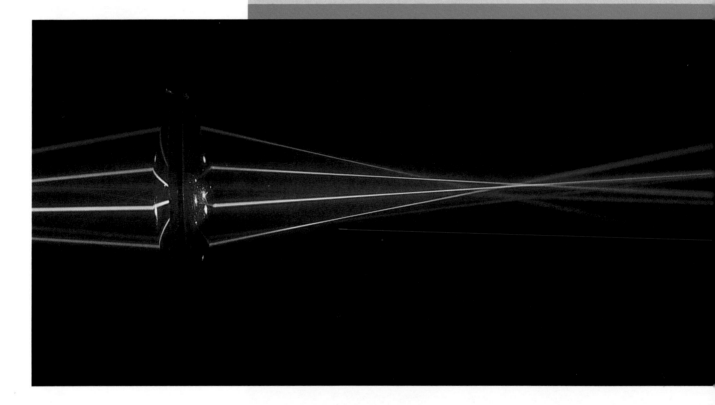

The evidence for that long mammalian night is found in the structure of their diurnal eye. When mammals returned to the daylight, blinking and tearing from the glare of the sun, they had lost the colored oil droplets found in more primitive vertebrates to protect their photoreceptors from ultraviolet damage and reduce their eye's most serious drawback, chromatic aberration.

Chromatic Abberation

While the vertebrate eye is significantly better at absorbing light and seeing over long distances than is the compound eye, it suffers from the blurring of the colors in the image on the retina. Of what use is to be able to see great distances if the blue and red part of an image are out of focus? Since wavelengths of light vary in energy, vibrating at different speeds, no vertebrate lens can bend all of them equally so that they strike the retina in one focal plane. The more energetic shorter wavelengths focus in front of the retina while the longer wavelengths are brought into focus behind it; the result, a blurred image. Without some help, the ciliary muscles of the eye would be constantly squeezing and stretching the lens without ever succeeding in forming a clear optical image. Worse, the vertebrate lens hardens with age, making it less malleable—as people over forty gradually become aware.

▲

Argon beams refracted through a lens. Because wavelengths vary in energy, no known lens can bend them so that they land at exactly the same point. This is one reason why human eyes suffer from color distortion.

Nature's solution was to sacrifice certain wavelengths by blocking them out and giving the lens less work to do. This means that some colors can no longer be seen. Normally it is the shorter wavelengths that are filtered since these are in the ultraviolet range and are also potentially harmful to visual tissue.

Filtering the Sun

The first filters were colored oil droplets found within the individual photoreceptors themselves. These selectively block wavelengths according to their own color. Some are shades of orange, others yellow; birds and turtles also have red oil droplets. Oil droplets are found even in primitive fish, such as the sturgeon, and amphibians, and there are clear oil droplets in the eyes of monotremes and marsupials.

Since nocturnal creatures need all the light they can get, their oil droplets either lost their coloration, which makes them totally ineffective at blocking any wavelengths of light, or completely disappeared. But when formerly nocturnal creatures re-emerged into the daylight, nature did not re-create the variously colored oil droplets, which by the way give birds a far more varied color picture of the world than our own, but replaced them instead with an all-encompassing yellow filter that completely fills the lens. Some mammals, including ourselves, have a second yellow filter covering the cone-rich fovea. Mammals share this type of filter with modern teleost fish and the snake, which lost its legs as well as its oil droplets when it burrowed underground.

The Structure of the Diurnal Mammalian Eye

Smaller in proportion to body size than the nocturnal mammalian eye, the eye of the diurnal mammal retains the major advance found in the eye of the bird; the lens is pushed forward toward the cornea, increasing the size of the image that falls on the retina. The eye is protected by an outer layer called the sclera, part of which we refer to as the "white" of the eye. Next comes the cornea, which has the primary responsibility for focusing light on the retina of land vertebrates; some

mammals, in fact, do not have any lens accommodation at all, relying only on the cornea for a visual image. The iris opens or shuts depending on the amount of light available, and the structure of the eye is sustained by two jellylike layers: the aqueous and vitreous humor.

Most mammalian retinas are duplex, that is, containing both rods and cones passing on their visual information to neural cells: first the bipolars, then the ganglion, and thence, via the optic nerve, to the brain. Additional neural cells, the amacrine and horizontal cells, participate in the forwarding or inhibiting of visual information and may even have the responsibility of wiping the visual slate clean. Six sturdy ocular muscles move the eye about, keeping it in constant motion, voluntary and involuntary, so that individual photoreceptors have time to revitalize themselves with forms of Vitamin A_1 and A_2 while others fire. Behind the retina is a blood-rich layer that provides the retina's nourishment (the choroid layer).

Animals are rarely aware of this network of blood vessels unless light strikes their eyes from a particular angle; you might have become aware of your own if an ophthalmologist or optometrist has ever shined a light into your eyes.

Most wild animals are emmetropic, that is, normally sighted or

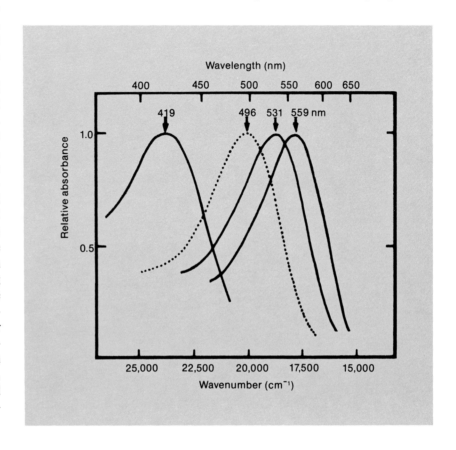

Human retinal cones are most sensitive to wavelengths of 419, 531 and 559 nm (solid curves), while rods are most sensitive to wavelengths of 496 nm (dotted curve). Our best color discrimination occurs where the cone curves overlap.

even somewhat farsighted, while domesticated creatures, such as guinea pigs, rabbits and even chickens, are generally nearsighted. (Those of us who wear glasses may well want to ponder this fact.) Life in a hutch or pen can cause a change in visual attention, which can affect the range of vision.

The Chiasma—The Optic Crossroads

Two completely new developments occurred in the vision of mammals: consensual pupillary movements (this means that both pupils widen or get smaller at the same time) and coordinated eye movements. Both are the result of increased facility of visuomotor organization (visual commands made to the eyes by the brain).

In all sub-mammalian species, including marsupials and monotremes, the visual information from the left eye crosses over to the right hemisphere of the brain and the information from the right eye crosses over to the left hemisphere; the vision science term for this is *complete decussation*. But in primitive mammals we see the beginnings of a new development; some of the visual channels in the optic nerve split off and go to the same eye. As a result, each hemisphere gets information from both eyes.

The percentage of information going to the same hemisphere varies in different creatures: in the dog it's ¼; in the cat, ⅓; in the horse, ⅙ to ⅛. By the time we reach the primates, the split has become 50 percent.

The split of information at the chiasma is responsible ultimately for one of the more remarkable aspects of mammalian and, in particular, primate vision—three-dimensional stereoscopic vision. Splitting the visual information at the chiasma improves depth perception. The corpus callosum, which is the link that connects the two hemispheres of the mammalian brain, makes it possible for the brain to compare the two disparate retinal images of each eye. One of the ways the brain judges distance is ocular convergence, comparing the angle between the sighted object and each eye. The movement of the ocular muscles as the object is brought into focus helps the brain judge the exact distance. Furthermore, as the distance between an object and an

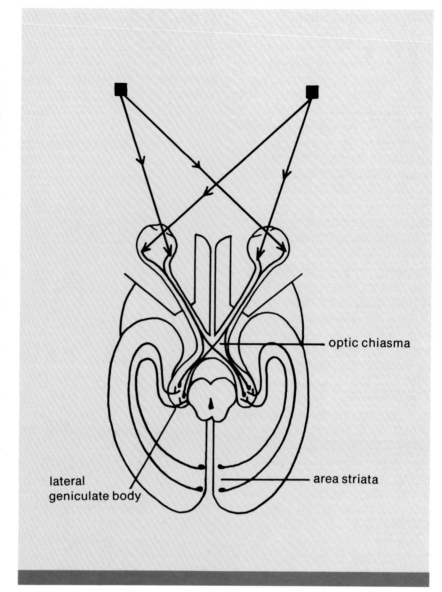

optic chiasma

lateral geniculate body

area striata

▲

Chiasma, or optic crossroads. In more primitive creatures, all information from each eye goes to the opposite side of the brain. But in mammals, instead of crossing completely at the optic chiasma, the optic nerve also sends some of its fibers to the same side. In primates, this split is 50 percent, enabling them to compare images from each eye with split-second rapidity and forming the basis for stereoscopic depth perception.

animal increases, the pupils widen to let in more light. All this requires extensive coordination between the sensory-motor system and the visual system, sometimes called the visuomotor system.

As we ascend the mammalian evolutionary ladder, this type of coordination becomes more complex. The behavior of lower mammals is still largely instinctual; some of the visual cells in the eyes of the rabbit, for example, trigger certain kinds of behavior directly. But as creatures evolve, the number of responses an animal can make in a given situation increases logarithmically. Thought, the comparing of alternatives, is in-

volved, and that takes time. It becomes absolutely necessary for both hemispheres of the brain to receive visual information from both eyes as quickly as possible.

Protecting the Eye—
Open and Closed Orbits

The eye is the only direct opening of the central nervous system to the world, and nature has evolved different types of skull enclosures to protect it. The oldest is the closed orbit, which is found in primates including ourselves; one can feel the bones of our temples and cheeks joining to enclose our eyes. Open orbits are a comparatively modern innovation though, by nature's standards, modern means several million years ago. Skulls with open orbits do not completely enclose the eye, and there is a large triangular section extending back over the temples that is not covered by bone. Among carnivores there is a strange correlation between open orbits and the ability of a creature to open its mouth wide. The saber-toothed tiger was the clear champion, having been able to open its mouth to an angle of 90 degrees; but then, it lived in an age of giant mammals. Birds also have open orbits, with the exception of the Australian cockatoo. Since the eyes of birds have become larger at the expense of their brains, nature has obviously tried to give them every possible bit of space to expand. Open orbits are also found in amphibians and marsupials.

There are species that started out with open orbits but evolved to closed orbits; one such example is the horse. The reason should be obvious: Stallions fight, causing terrible damage to each other with their teeth and hooves, and an overall skull gives far more protection.

Range of Vision

The question that seems to invite the curiosity of most people is whether or not their pet can see in color. Thus good form vision is assumed, though range of vision and acuity vary widely among mammals. Most mammals have a fixed-focal-length lens and lack the ciliary muscles that alter the lens' shape for near or far vision, though smaller mammals with a short-focal-length lens have an extremely large depth of field and can see great distances.

In land vertebrates, the cornea bears the primary responsibility for focusing light on the retina; its index of refraction is greater than that of any other medium in the eye, including the lens. In more advanced land mammals, the lens is suspended by zonular fibers that attach to the ciliary muscles. The zonular fibers contract for near vision and relax for far vision. Looking off into the distance is more relaxing to the vertebrate eye than looking at something close. Most vision scientists believe that the avian and reptilian lens systems are better engineered than the mammal's because they rely on greater effort of the muscles rather than the elasticity of the lens, which hardens with age.

There is a correlation between an animal's ability to reach out and grasp an object (praxic skill) and the development of lens accommodation. The more an animal is able to manipulate its environment, the greater the potential for lens accommodation. During the long period of nocturnality, mammals who lived in trees developed hands and feet for grasping limbs and even small insects—the earliest primates were insectivores—as well as the musculature to squeeze the lens. Their visual attention required quick changes in focus, and eye-hand coordination became of paramount importance. Of mammals that remained on the ground, only those who used their paws with any consistency developed any sort of lens accommodation at all. The rabbit, for example, has no lens accommodation whatsoever; the dog's is limited to one diopter. (The diopter is a measure of distance over which an eye can see clearly, equal to one meter.) Cats use their paws more than most other animals, and their focal range is considerably larger, from about 3.5D to 11.5D. But the otter and the beaver have the greatest range of any creatures with paws; it is significant that they are master builders and must also contend with the change in refraction between air and water. These creatures have unusually large sphincter muscles in their iris to squeeze the lens as well as strong ciliary muscles.

Color Vision in
Mammals

Perhaps the variations in human color vision can help us to better understand the color vision of animals. We refer to some people as color blind even though all normal human beings are certainly color blind in the near-ultraviolet accessible to most insects as well as the near-infrared seen by freshwater fish such as the perch. Monochromats are completely color blind and see the world in shades of gray, black and white. Either their retinas lack cones completely or the cones do not function properly. This is a comparatively rare condition in humans but a common one in animals. Dichromats see the world in shades of blues and yellows and are blind in either the red or green area of the spectrum. This is the most common form of human color blindness but is in fact the way that many animals see. Dichromats' retinas always have short-wavelength cones but lack either medium-wavelength cones or long-wavelength cones. The tritanope cannot distinguish colors in the short-wavelength area of the spectrum. This is a rare condition in humans and is produced by illness or injury rather than genetic defect. Furthermore, this type of condition has never been found in animals.

The first cones to evolve were medium-wavelength cones, which served simply as luminosity or brightness detectors.

The second to evolve was the short-wavelength cone. It is interesting to speculate on why nature chose the blue or even blue-violet area of the spectrum. Perhaps it was because we evolved out of the sea, where only short wavelengths of light can penetrate to any depth. Then, finally, came the long-wavelength cone, which animals use to spot ripening fruits and berries and even danger markings on poisonous creatures, as well as our dramatic red sunsets (made more glorious by current pollution).

Each cone has a wavelength maximum, but it also may have a secondary peak (see illustration). These peaks overlap, and it is within the area of overlap that the animal can best compare differences in wavelengths, or what appears to the eye as differences in color. Two cones give limited color vision, and three cones allow for what is called normal trichromatic vision, though there can be variations from eye to eye, even from human eye to eye.

The color vision of the dichromatic animal varies widely from normal trichromatic vision. Imagine a world where reds appear dark brown and there is a large area in the middle of the spectrum called a neutral point which you couldn't distinguish from white. This normally falls in the frequency of what appears to us as green. The quality of what color vision they have may also be more limited.

Dichromats compare short and medium wavelength radiation. The short wavelength cone is far more susceptible to disease and trauma than other cones, and it contributes very little to perceiving spatial boundaries or luminosity. There are few of them in foveas and none at all in the central region of the fovea. Dichromatic animals must rely on their rod vision for spatial and temporal resolution, but rods do not function in bright sunlight. It is possible, then, that theirs is not only a blue and yellow world but often a somewhat fuzzy blue and yellow world. In addition, the dichromat requires far more light to distinguish the same colors that can be seen by both dichromat and tri-

chromat; as much as ten times more light may be required.

Vision scientists know more about some animals than others. Behavioral studies are rarely performed on crocodiles or the fierce Tasmanian devil; rabbits, rats, cats, monkeys, goldfish and pigeons appear to be the preferred sources of information, but more is being discovered every day. What follows is a brief survey of some of what has been learned.

The Cat

The cat has been a companion to man since pharaonic Egypt if not before. As such, it became more diurnal in its habits, but many cats nevertheless sleep much of the day away and prowl at night. The evidence of the cat's early nocturnality shimmers in the golden glow of its tapetum, which increases the light available for vision. The cat's is a tapetum fibrosum, which is not as reflective as that of the fish, which is made from guanine, the same substance found in scales. But it is the most common type of tapetum in animals and is located in the choroid coat just beyond the retina. Animals with this type of tapetum have highly contractile pupils that they close during the day. The cat pupil appears circular when open but contracts to a narrow slit in bright light.

For some time it was assumed that cats had no color vision. Since they're such an independent lot it is difficult to design behavioral experiments for them, but there is now evidence that they have a middle and short wavelength cone but no long cone. All evidence suggests that the cat is a dichromat with vision similar to a human being who is red-green blind. What appears red to us is simply dark to the cat, and a part of the green spectrum is indistinguishable from white, though the neutral points

vary for each dichromat.

What is more, the evidence also suggests that the cat's color vision is mediated by its rods as well as its cones. The cat's color vision is best under what is known as mesopic conditions, when the sunlight is not as strong, during the early morning or late afternoon. (In brilliant sunlight, the rods cease to function, and since cats have so few cones, their vision is very poor in bright light.) Since rods and cones use the same neural pathways, when they are both activated the result should be a desaturation of the color signal. Colors that would appear very rich to us are more pastel-like to the cat. Does this mean when the cat walks on a green, grassy lawn past a bush of red roses that what it sees is a whitish lawn and a whitish bush with dark flowers? The answer is most probably yes.

Cats have about six times fewer cones in their retinas than we do, only about 25,000 per square millimeter. While cats do not have a round fovea, the section of highest photoreceptor concentration is known as the area centralis, which is less specific in shape.

The cornea of the cat is larger and more curved than the human cornea, perhaps to make up for the limited accommodative power of its lens. Refractive errors are rare in cats, but when they do occur, the cat is generally nearsighted. Generally the cat's vision is best about six to eighteen feet in front of it. Most carnivores have their eyes positioned slightly more in front of their face, but the domestic cat has an angle of between five to ten degrees between its eyes. Thus it has a wider field of vision, about 210 degrees compared to our own field of vision of only about 140 degrees. Is it possible that the cat's angle of vision has widened since its domestication because it no longer needs the strong binocular vision of the predator?

The Siamese Cat

Despite their obvious intelligence, there is something a little spacey about the gaze of a Siamese cat. A mutation in its genes that is also responsible for this cat's characteristic coat color causes the optic nerves to make a complete cross at the optic chiasma. In this respect, the Siamese cat is a throwback to sub-mammalian species. Since information from each eye goes only to the opposite hemisphere of the brain, it has no stereoscopic vision and is forced to make judgments concerning depth using only monocular cues.

The eye of the cat is rod-dominated with few cone receptors. In bright light, when rod receptors cease to function, the cat's slit pupil shuts almost completely, keeping most of the light out of the eye and allowing the rods to continue to operate.

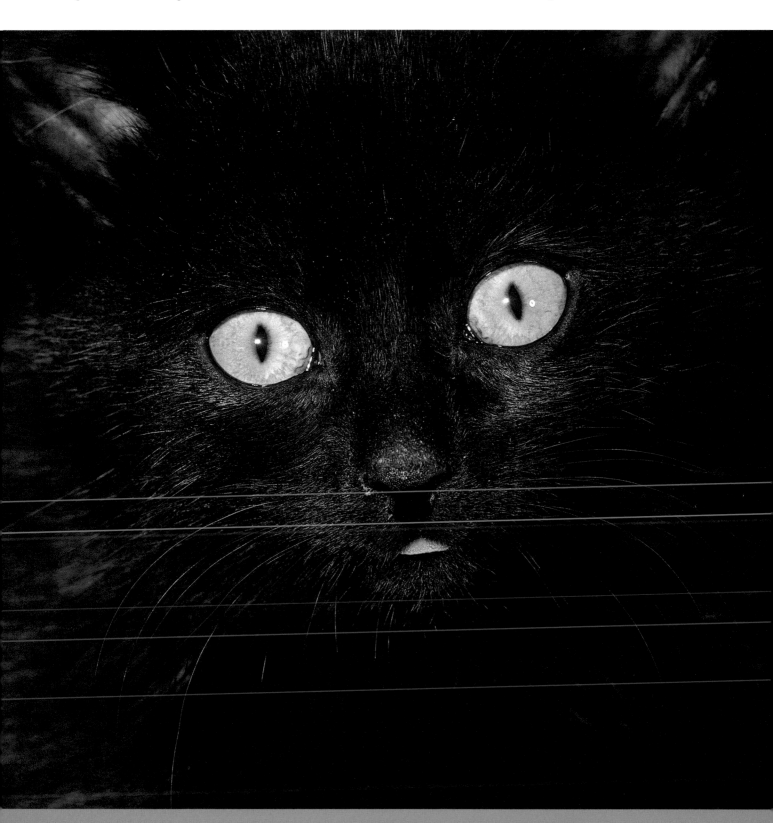

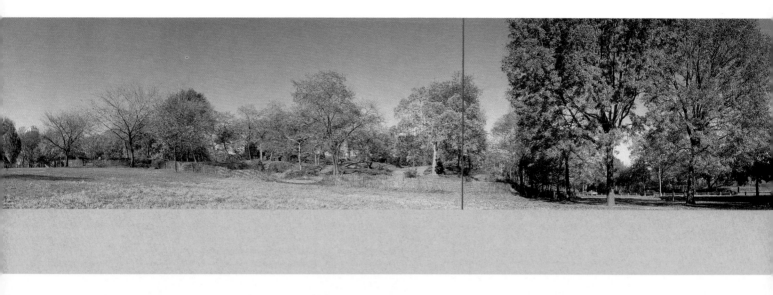

The Cheetah

The cheetah is the only large wild cat that is diurnal. It is a solitary hunter and the fastest carnivore alive. To protect its eyes from the glare of the African sun, nature has added a circle of black fur under each eye. While no studies of color vision are available for this creature, it is reasonable to assume that its vision resembles that of the domestic cat. Range of vision is another question, and the cheetah, which has larger eyes, may even be somewhat farsighted.

The Rabbit

The rabbit has a truly panoramic view of the world, a nearly 360-degree field of vision. In fact, its eyes are so widely separated that it has a large blind spot directly in front of it. Even if the rabbit's brain compensates, it is possible that the image it sees is somewhat distorted, like an extremely wide-angle photograph. While the rabbit has a wide field of vision, its binocular overlap is limited to about 10 to 34 degrees. This means that it has very little depth perception.

The rabbit has a most primitive mammalian brain, with an almost nonexistent neocortex. Sixty percent of the rabbit's receptor fields are selective, meaning that they respond to specific features of visual images. Selectivity is not good for form discrimination but good for telling size or location. In higher mammals, the development of selective responses is delayed till the visual cortex. The rabbit's brain is so primitive that it can lose most of its neocortex and still detect light and movement and pos-

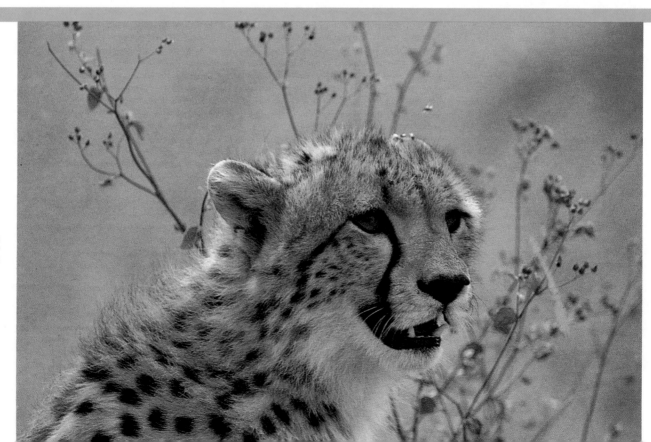

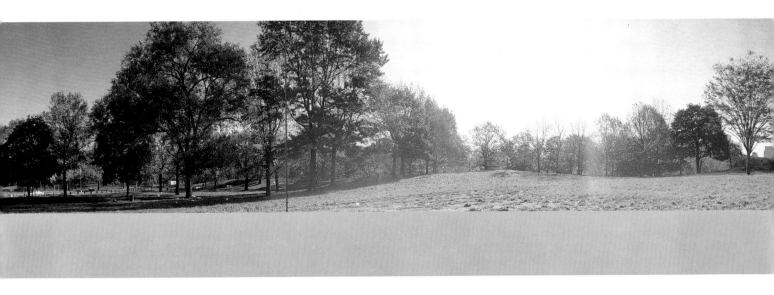

sibly even retain some form vision. It is a creature that still sees with its eyes, unlike more advanced mammals who "see" with their brains.

The rabbit has a fixed-focus lens with no accommodation. When frightened, it simply freezes and does not even attempt to follow the predator with its eyes. Certainly it has no means of defending itself, so that flight or freeze are its only solutions. Its greatest asset is its ability to see so much of what is going on around it on the chance that what it might see means trouble.

The Dog

There are more than 300 breeds of dogs—short dogs and tall dogs, dogs with tails and without, dogs with eyes that bulge out of their heads like the Pekinese and little beasts that are almost blinded by the hair that covers them.

We know that dogs have a smaller visual range than we do, far less lens accommodation than the cat. Refractive errors in the eye of dogs are limited and when they exist are rarely above two diopters. While the

human eye is larger, the dog's lens is much bigger, perhaps to compensate for its lack of accommodative power.

Dogs do not have a fovea, though they may have a rod-rich concentration of photocells with a limited number of cones. For a long time it was thought that dogs had absolutely no color vision, but current thinking is that they do have limited color vision. The dog is probably a dichromat with a total inability to distinguish reds and greens. It can see comparatively few colors and only those in the short wavelength area, the

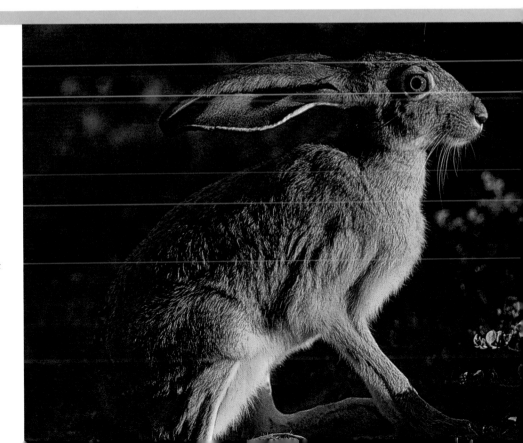

▲ ▶

The eyes of the rabbit are placed so far back on the sides of its head that it has almost 360-degree vision all around but a comparatively large blind spot dead ahead. This picture taken with a panoramic camera gives us some idea of the extent of the rabbit's visual fields. The red lines show where the human visual fields end, at about 140 degrees.

The cheetah is the only large diurnal predatory cat. Nature has given it black circles under its eyes to absorb some of the daylight glare.

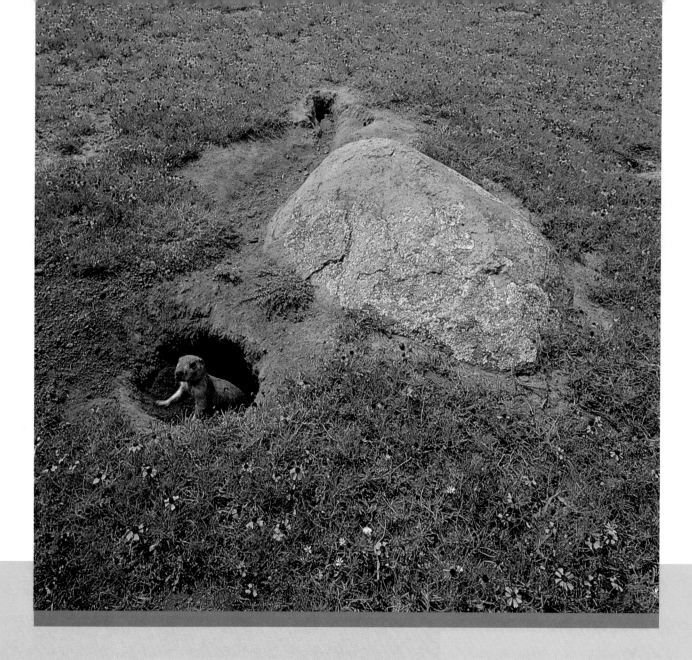

▲ ▲

Red-green blindness occurs only rarely in human beings, but it is the norm for many animals. Squirrels and prairie dogs, for example, cannot distinguish reds, and green appears to them as neutral as white. Compared to ours, theirs is a blue-and-yellow world.

blues, with any consistency.

Even with limited visual range, it has good form perception, and experiments show that it can even discriminate certain basic shapes, such as an ellipse from a circle.

The Prairie Dog and the Squirrel

It should be somewhat obvious from their appearance that these two creatures are related, and they certainly share visual similarities. These two members of the class Sciuridae are the only mammals to have cone-rich retinas. In fact, for a time it was thought that they had only cones in their retinas, but since the advent of the electron microscope a number of rod photoreceptors have been recognized, though not enough to play any role in their vision. Like the turtle, which also has a cone-rich retina, both are almost blind at night.

There is no doubt that both the squirrel and the prairie dog have color vision. Both are dichromats, lacking a long wavelength cone, and see the world in shades of blues and yellows. Blue skies and yellow sand are all quite well for the prairie dog, since there is little green in the desert; but what of the squirrel, who lives amid the forest greenery, little of which is

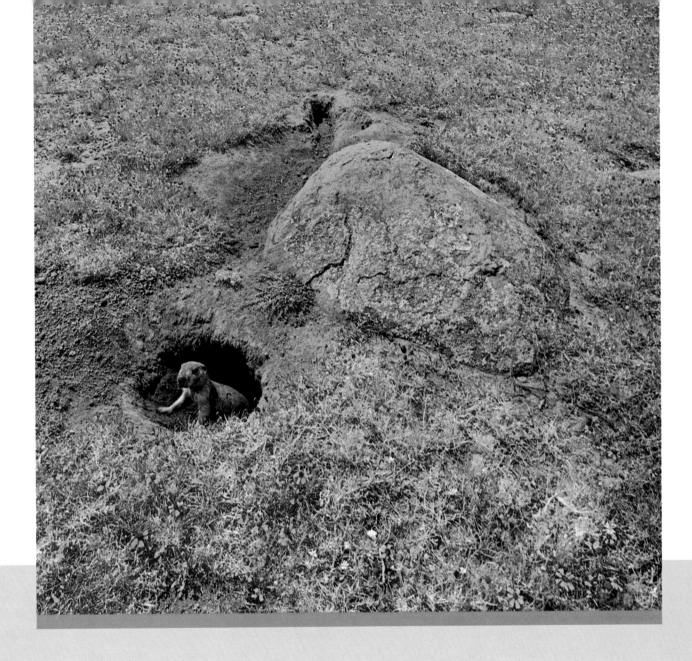

accessible to its vision because the dichromatic neutral point is found in the green area of the spectrum?

The prairie dog can see in light that would make human eyes blink and tear. We know that the dichromat requires more light to distinguish the colors it can see, and in the desert it certainly gets it. Prairie dogs are social creatures, and several are always on guard in their communal towns standing above the burrows. They constantly scan the horizon for intruders, and should one be spotted, they give a loud warning whistle,

which brings the other prairie dogs out. Then all stand and watch till the intruder either disappears or comes too close, waiting until the last moment to disappear into the safety of their burrows. Such playfulness and courage may indicate a high level of intelligence.

The eyes of the squirrel protrude from its head, and like the rabbit, some species have an almost 360-degree panoramic view of the world, though most end at 320°. These creatures are normally sighted, and refractive errors are rare. The use of their

paws to pick up nuts and other objects indicates that they have some degree of lens accommodation. Considering that they can see almost completely around their heads, their protruding eyes give them a surprisingly high degree of binocularity, about 25 to 30 degrees. The yellow filter of the squirrel tends to be darker than that of other mammals; perhaps the cone-rich retina requires more protection. In general, the yellow filters of mammals living in warmer climates tend to be darker than those farther from the equator.

Rats and Mice

About 40 percent of rodents are nocturnal. Those who are not exhibit some degree of color vision, though they do not appear to be able to distinguish hues separated by less than 50nm, while we know that the human eye can distinguish colors separated by only 1nm in some parts of the spectrum. Other mammals with color vision can generally discriminate colors separated by 20nm, so you can see that rodents' color vision is not very good.

Rats are a favorite subject for vision scientists, and one bit of intriguing, though as yet unexplained, information learned from psychological experimentation is that rats prefer mazes that exhibit regular patterns over those that are random.

The Horse

Normally we associate the movement of a horse's head with spirited behavior. But if classical vision theory is correct, it is not just vitality that causes the head to bob about but a need to properly focus an image on different sections of its retina. The horse is reputed to have a ramp retina, that is, a retina that is not equidistant from the lens but is tilted forward from the bottom. If George Walls is correct in *The Vertebrate Eye*, the horse shares this peculiarity with a creature that bears no resemblance to it whatsoever, the marine ray.

Walls suggests that the ramp retina is a compensation for lack of musculature to change the shape of the horse's lens, so that it accommodates for near and far vision by the movement of its head, directing the image to a suitable part of the retina. The head goes down for far vision and up for close, though it sees the ground clearly when it is grazing because of the natural slope of its head.

This is a major reason for giving the horse some freedom of head

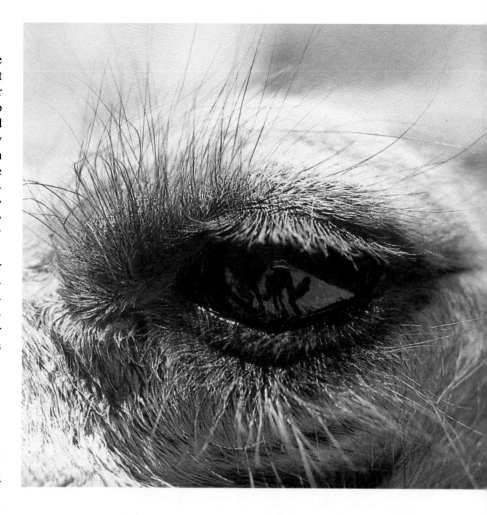

▲
The camel is one of the few large vertebrates that still has a nictitating membrane, which it draws over the eye during sandstorms.

movement when riding. When moving swiftly, it sees clearly only at a distance; for example, it is blind to a jump when it gets about four feet away from it.

Some modern vision scientists challenge the idea of the ramp retina, and a fairly recent Canadian study found no evidence of it in a large group of horses examined. Furthermore, the study found an area centralis in the retina, a high concentration of photoreceptors similar to a fovea, which the researchers maintain contradicts the idea of a ramp retina.

The horse has a wide visual field, of 190 to 195 degrees, and the transverse muscles of the eye in the nasal area can extend its visual field to 215 degrees. The horse can see behind itself in lines parallel to the axis of its body; hence the use of blinders on racehorses, to keep their concentration on what's in front of them.

Like other ungulates (herbivorous, hooved creatures), the horse develops horizontal astigmatism generally from its third year. The focus of the horse's vision is obviously the distant horizon.

Other Ungulates

The zebra has vision very much like the horse's, but it is worth mentioning separately because of the nature of the visual camouflage of its coat. The striping of the zebra stands out during the day, but the zebra has both good vision to warn it of approaching predators and the speed to escape. Not so at night; galloping in the dark, when most predators hunt, can be dangerous. The stripes or, as they are called in vision science, gratings, take advantage of a fundamental mechanism of image analysis in the vertebrate eye. It simply cannot analyze them in low light levels and so the zebra is almost undetectable from dusk to dawn.

Most ungulates have good acuity because their eyes are large and rod-rich, though there are exceptions. The hippo and the elephant have as few photoreceptors in the center of their eyes as we do in the periphery and are reputed to be able to see clearly for only about several hundred feet. Ungulates also tend to horizontal astigmatism from searching the horizon for predators.

The giraffe, on the other hand, can see the approach of a man at least two kilometers away. As befits a muncher of leaves of some height, its eyes face downward. The giraffe has also been tested for color vision and is able to distinguish some colors such as red and violet, though it confuses green, orange and yellow.

For many years it was widely assumed that ungulates simply had no color vision. Tests are difficult to organize, but it is becoming clear that, like other animals with a limited number of cones, many of these creatures see in color under medium light, when both rods and cones work together. A deer may not be able to see a hunter wearing an orange jacket in

▶

Some hunters are aware that deer have limited color vision, but only in relatively dim light. Like many creatures with few retinal cones, they require more light to discriminate changes in wavelength, so that in the early morning, they can only see in black and white. In bright light, when rods cannot function, they have too few cones to give them good vision.

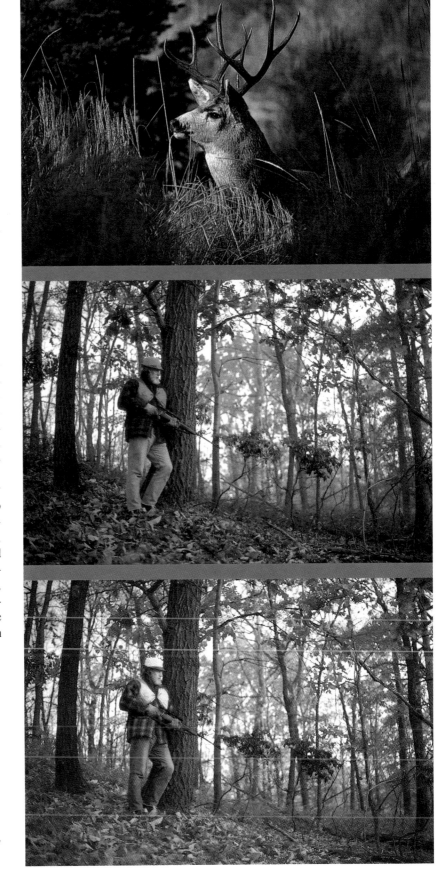

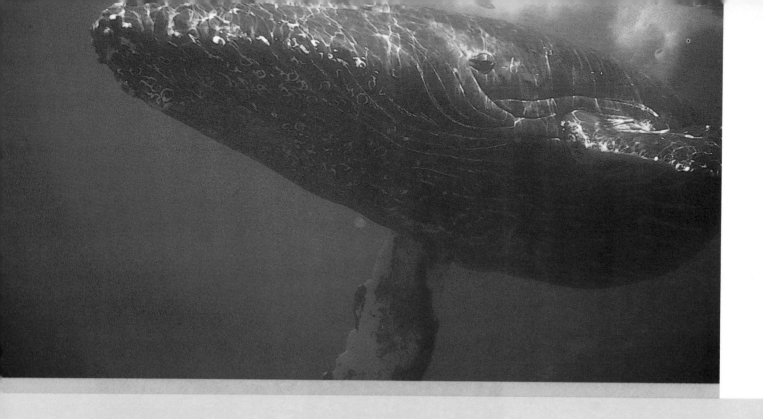

the early morning or late afternoon. Deer probably do not see well in bright sunlight. Like cats that have few cones, their vision suffers when their rods do not function. Even sheep are reputed to have some color vision. Many of them also still have tapeta and nictitating membranes, the vestiges of a once-nocturnal existence.

The Mammals of the Deep

Sixty-five million years ago something happened on earth that ultimately destroyed the great reptiles. Curiously it was also about that time that a species of mammals chose to return to life in the sea. These were the cetaceans: whales and dolphins. They were followed a few million years later by the sirenians (manatees and dugongs), gentle creatures who dwell in the coastal waters of the United States and Asia and who are sometimes mistaken for the mythical mermaid. Fifty million years later another species followed, seals and walruses (the pinnipeds).

Both cetaceans and sirenians have become so adapted to life in the sea that they remain there to breed, but the pinnipeds must return to land for that. The ecology of this behavior affects their vision; seals and walruses must be able to see well on land and in the water. Once again, corneas adapted for life in the sea make an animal extremely nearsighted on land. Yet seals are known to poke their heads out of water to examine a beach before coming ashore.

Nature has given these creatures a visual mechanism used before in reptiles such as the gecko. It is the stenopeic pupil, the slit pupil that can shut down on land to a pinhole opening. Of course the gecko does not have to contend with a change from aquatic to terrestrial life, as do the seal and the walrus, and the stenopeic pupil also requires a great deal of light. But at least they can see on land in daylight. In addition, their cornea is astigmatic along the horizontal axis, and what ordinarily would be a defect is

put to good use in their land vision since the astigmatism crosses the center of the stenopeic pupil, giving them even sharper vision.

Proof of the *Pinnipedia's* (it means ''fin-like feet'') earlier existence as a land creature is found in the fetus. During the first part of fetal development the eyes are clearly frontal like those of its carnivorous terrestrial ancestor, but before birth they move slowly to opposite sides of the head, increasing the field of vision.

A wide field of vision must be an important factor to survival in the water. In some whales it is carried to an extreme. The eyes of the sperm and blue whale, for example, have moved to completely opposite sides of the head. Whales have an enormous blind spot directly in front of them. They have absolutely no binocular vision. One of the techniques of whaling was for the ship to approach the whale from directly in front so that there was less chance of it being seen. Yet the sperm whale will lift its head out of water to get a better look,

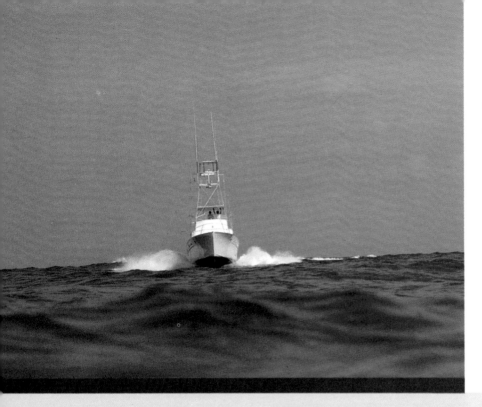

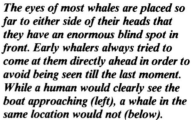

The eyes of most whales are placed so far to either side of their heads that they have an enormous blind spot in front. Early whalers always tried to come at them directly ahead in order to avoid being seen till the last moment. While a human would clearly see the boat approaching (left), a whale in the same location would not (below).

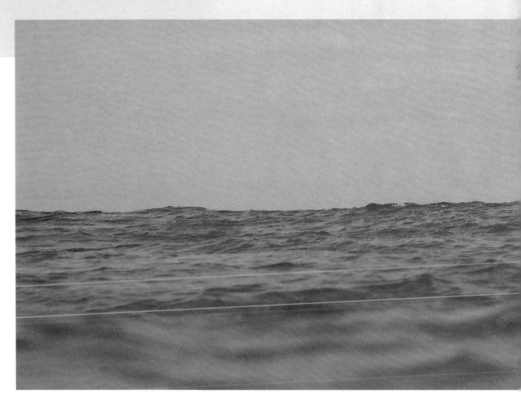

and bottleneck dolphins can see moving objects in the air at forty feet with their heads out of water. Smaller cetaceans such as dolphins use their eyesight to hunt fast-moving fish.

One of the reasons the eyes of whales are so small may be that the sclera, or covering of the eye, is subjected to enormous pressures when the whale dives. The sclera of the whale is unusually tough. The eyes of whales and dolphins are oval, with a large spherical lens. The whale's eyes face down toward the stomach, while the seal's eyes face upward. It all depends on the direction in which one searches for food. Certain seals are nocturnal feeders (Phocidae), and all seals' eyes are dark-adapted with a tapetum, though most seals are diurnal in habit. Bioluminescent fish and squid tend to rise at night to feed and become the seal's prey. On a moonlit night, the outline of a surface fish becomes visible from below. (The positioning of the seal's eyes explains why they are so good at catching fish thrown to them in the zoo.)

There are two types of whales,

the Odontoceti or toothed whales, which are flesh eaters, and the baleen whale. The eyesight of the baleen whale is not as good as that of the toothed whale because these giant creatures do not search for food as much as trawl, siphoning in krill and other tiny crustaceans in enormous

quantities. They are the largest creatures on earth, particularly the blue and sperm whales—larger than any dinosaur. The dinosaur's body had to support itself on land, as their enormous skeletons attest, but every inch of the whale's body is supported by the uplift of water.

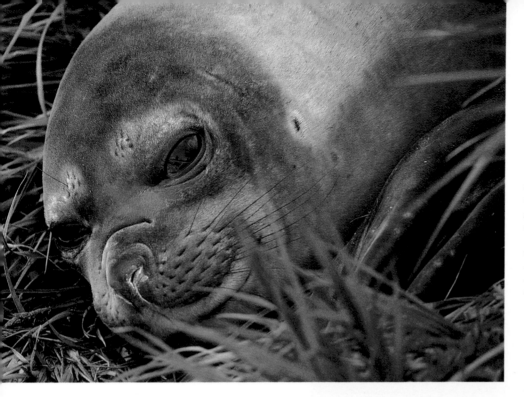

◀ ▼

The seal and walrus returned to life in the water several million years after the cetaceans, and while their eyes have progressively moved to the sides of their heads, this is still not as marked as in whales and dolphins. In fact, the eyes of the seal fetus are directly in front, much like its land ancestor of millennia before, and they only move to the side of the head shortly before birth.

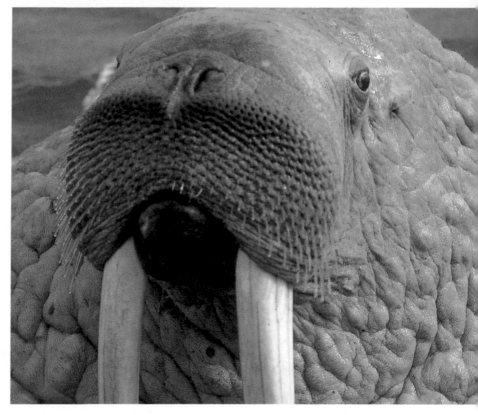

Since they lack stenopoeic pupils, their eyesight cannot be as good as that of the seal out of water, yet toothed whales such as the killer whale are known to check ice floes for prey. But the downward tilt of the whale eye is evidence that their favorite food is the giant squid. Whales have no eyelids or lachrymal glands but secrete an oily substance that coats their eyes, eyes by the way that never shut, even in sleep.

The importance of the brain in mammalian vision is a given. The increased size of the neocortex in mammals, primates and subsequently man is responsible for the complexity of the visuomotor system. If the neocortex is important to the vision of the land mammal, the extraordinary size of the cortex in whales and dolphins, so much larger than our own, suggests that it might compensate somewhat for the smallness of their eyes and the difficult medium in which these creatures must see.

The eyes of the Asian dugong and American manatee are much like the human eye, though the ciliary muscles in these *Sirenia* are vestigial

and they have no lens accommodation for near and far vision. These creatures, as should be expected, are normally sighted in water and nearsighted in air, though they rarely poke their heads above the surface. When they do, vision makes them particularly vulnerable to the blades of motorboats.

These shy vegetarians have eyes that are nocturnally adapted yet lack all remnants of a tapetum. Living so close to the surface may give them sufficient light. While there are some cones in their retinas, there is no evidence for color vision.

13 *Primates*

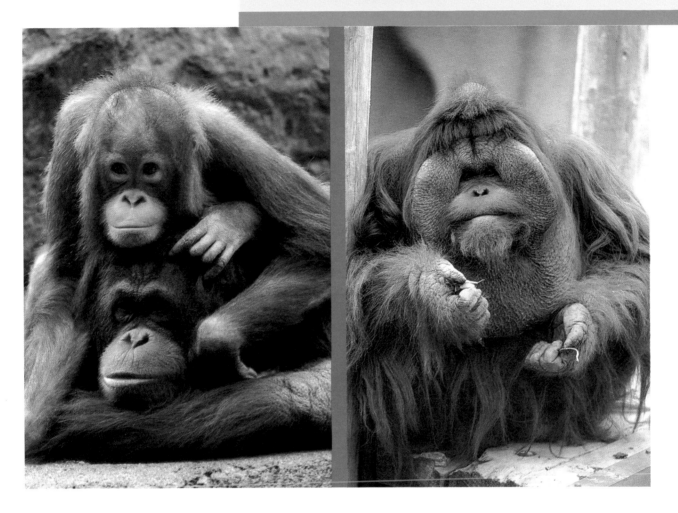

I t should come as no surprise that the vision of many primates closely resembles our own, though some scientists insist that molecular biology shows we are evolutionarily twice as close to African apes such as the chimpanzee and the gorilla than Asian apes such as the gibbon and the orangutan.

There is no doubt that life in the trees had a salutary effect on the evolution of the primate's vision. It is certain that the hand designed for grasping and holding evolved simultaneously with the musculature nec-essary to change the shape of the lens for near and far vision, an ability that we use to dramatic effect in our own lives, from playing tennis to piloting a complex aircraft.

The earliest arboreal mammals, from which the primates emerged, depended as much on their sense of smell as on their vision. But the change is evident in a creature close enough to the primates to be considered an evolutionary bridge, the tree shrew, *Tupaia glis*. Small, with a shrunken snout and large eyes, this nocturnal creature already has some

▲

Male orangutans seem to develop an especially thick skull as they mature. This one, in contrast to the female and juvenile, has a large bony plate around its head that limits its visual field.

color vision and limited depth per-ception. The lemur of Madagascar also has some color vision and is the only existing diurnal prosimian, having been protected by the wall of water that surrounds its island home from the more aggressive African and Asian simians. Yet it is in monkeys, chimps, baboons and gorillas that we find the greatest similarities to our own vision.

With the primate, we have come to that moment in evolution when how well an eye sees depends on the head in which it is found. For a primate sees with its brain as well as with its eyes.

We know from ablation studies (removal of various sections of the brain) that a primate may have a perfectly good eye and still lose its sight because of damage to the visual cortex; this is called blind sight. These discoveries were reinforced by the work of doctors on brain-damaged soldiers during both world wars. Parts of the visual field were no longer visible because of damage to a specific region of the visual cortex. What is even more interesting, some of the patients were not aware of the loss, much as we are unaware of our own blind spots unless they are pointed out to us. The brain suppresses the gap. While the increasing specialization of the cortex for vision and perception in primates has given us and the great apes an extraordinarily rich image of the world we live in such specialization can also hold a trap, for if a system fails, the result is blindness. The danger is less for monkeys, who can lose a significant portion of the neocortex and still use another section of the brain, the superior colliculus, to make out objects (though they will lose their texture).

What we call the superior colliculus is the entire brain available to more primitive creatures such as fish, amphibians, reptiles and birds. In these creatures it is known as the optic tectum. It appears that the neocortex of the mammal has been grafted onto this more ancient brain; in fact, it is even sometimes referred to as our "reptilian brain." Only the primate and the deep-sea cetacean (whales and dolphins) have a well-developed neocortex; indeed, the neocortex of the cetacean is far larger than our own.

The complexities of the neocortex have only begun to reveal themselves to science. We know that its organization is columnar; that is, cells are layered on top of one another. Walls in *The Vertebrate Eye* compares this organization to a geodesic map with one layer devoted to geography, another to topography, another to agriculture, and so on. But the brain is concerned not only with organizing the sensory information that comes to it but with making a response. At this point, we know more about the visual portion of the brain concerned with afferent channels— information that comes to it—than about the visuomotor system—visual responses directed by the brain. But it appears that many of the visuomotor responses (pupils of both eyes widening or diminishing at the same time and coordinated eye movements) are associated with the older brain, the superior colliculus.

More intriguing is the discovery by vision science that the organization of the brain mimics the cellular organization of the eye. The eye is constantly referred to as a minibrain. It is noted over and over again that the vertebrate eye is an "outgrowth" of the brain, yet the complex cellular organization of the eye preceded that of the brain.

Visual responses of primates differ from those of more primitive creatures in that they are mediated by the neocortex rather than being triggered by cells in the eye. Pigeons, it is said, can distinguish between different photographs more swiftly than human beings, so there is something to be said for the speed of trigger responses. But in the primate, the eye primarily transmits information to the brain, where the complexities of response are infinitely greater.

The eye of the primate is very similar to that of other mammals. Cells do not operate singly but in concert with other cells. Many receptors may affect a particular nerve cell at a different level of the visual system; the part of the visual field viewed by this collection of receptors is called the *receptor field* of the nerve cell. These receptor fields also exist for cells within the brain itself, but have a special character in the neocortex. Here the organization changes to a complex columnar layering where information from other sensory input frequently overlaps.

Where visual behavior is triggered by responses in the eye, we describe the receptive fields as being selective. The rabbit has a very small neocortex and at least 40 percent, if not more, of its receptive fields are described as being selective, while most of the receptive fields in the primate eye are non-selective, primarily transmitting information on to the neocortex.

One thing we do know is that color and form are analyzed separately; color vision is established within the eye itself, while form is the work of the visual cortex. Color vision theorists believe that much processing of color information is completed at the ganglion-cell level within the eyes, while form information is only finally synthesized in the visual cortex. This should not obscure the incredible specificity of cells in the visual cortex to color in a particular area of the visual field, indeed to a specific color in a particular area of the visual field; but the quality of the hue has already been established within the eye itself.

Color Vision in Primates

All primates have some color vision. The macaque has a color system of cone photoreceptors that closely matches our own. The wavelength maximums of the cones (short, medium and long receptors) are about the same as ours: 419nm, 531nm, 559nm, with the rods at 496nm. But if we examine these wavelength maximums very closely, we will discover that the long-wavelength receptor's maximum falls in the greenish-yellow area of the spectrum. A peculiar aspect of the primate trichromatic system is that it has no red receptor per se. The long-wavelength cone of the primate has its maximum absorption in the area of the spectrum that most closely matches the color of the forest canopy, greenish-yellow, a legacy from our earliest arboreal ancestors. How then do primates see red? Humans see red, and chimps and monkeys are known to spontaneously organize colored chips according to hue, including red, without any prompting. How did we go from creatures who could perceive only the greens and yellows of the forest to those who stop for red lights and wave red flags in front of bulls (which by the way, the bulls can't distinguish from any other dark color)?

The answer lies in the processing of the visual information by the nerve cells in the eye and ultimately the brain. The optical image that appears on the retina is only a part of the story. Even though the maximum sensitivity of the long-wavelength cone is 559nm, some of its visual pigment can absorb wavelengths above that, into the orange and red area of the spectrum. These wavelengths are also converted into energy and passed on to the next layer of cells, the bipolars. It is here that the transformation takes place.

The bipolar cells also have a maximum wavelength sensitivity, but theirs differs from that of the outer cone photoreceptors. Their activity shifts the eye's wavelength sensitivity and makes it possible for the primate eye to see red. Remember that the vertebrate eye is the only sensory organ that is an outgrowth of the brain. Each vertebrate eye is a processor as well as a receiver, with many more outer photoreceptors than nerve cells passing the visual information to the brain. Much of what the eye sees it transforms.

▶

The mandrill, like most other Old World monkeys, has color vision that resembles our own. In contrast, the primates of the New World have much more limited color vision.

Opponent Color Theory

After the photoreceptors convert light energy into chemical energy, it is passed successively to the bipolar and then to the ganglion cells. Horizontal and amacrine cells contribute to the passage or inhibition of color information before it is sent on to the brain.

Opponent color theory states that there are areas in successive parts of the eye and brain that are divided into receptive fields. Within these

fields there is a center group of cells that has one wavelength maximum that is directly opposed to the wavelength maximum of the group of cells that surround it: the center-surround. Cells responsive to wavelengths in the red area of the spectrum inhibit responses from wavelengths in the green area of the spectrum. Cells responsive to wavelengths in the blue area of the spectrum inhibit responses in the yellow area of the spectrum. Mirror groups of cells behave in just the reverse, and though the two systems

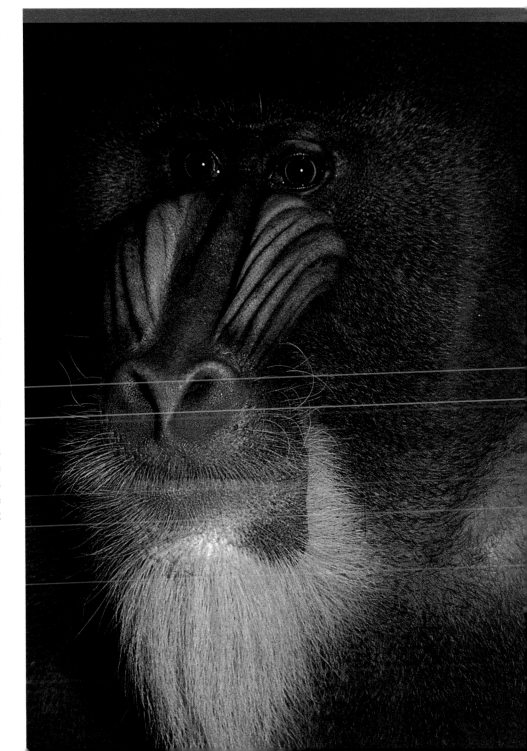

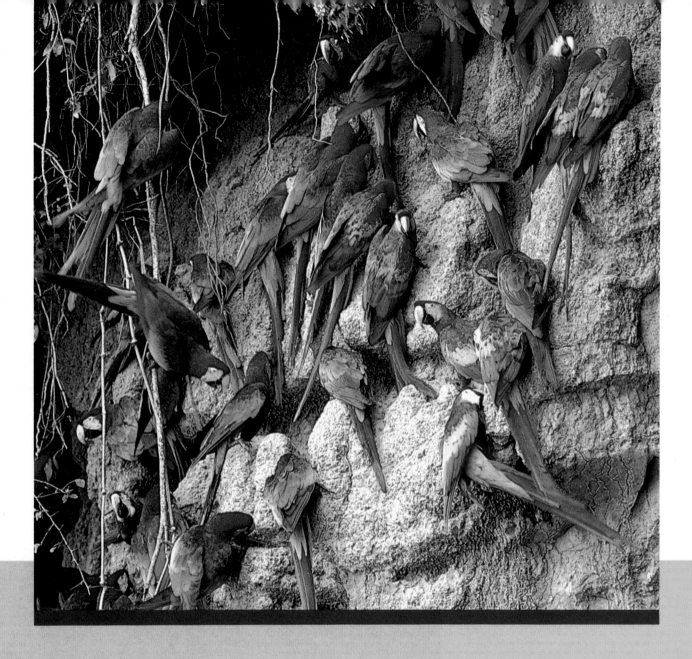

appear redundant, nature apparently takes few chances.

Primates with both systems are considered to have normal trichromatic systems; those without the red/green systems are known as dichromats. (It is not my intention to go into the history of color theory from Newton through Hering, Young, Hemholtz, et al., here as it is well covered in many other books.)

How is it that we can speak of four opponent colors (red/green, blue/yellow) when there are only three cone photoreceptors? It is important to note that there are no red, yellow, blue or green cone photoreceptors, only short-, medium-, and long-wavelength cones. Input from the long-wavelength cone signals red in the red/green system and yellow in the blue/yellow system. The medium-wavelength cone signals green in the red/green system and yellow in the blue/yellow system. In fact, we see pure yellow only when input into the red/green system balances out each of these colors. The permutations of only three cones are responsible for the wide variety of colors perceived by the primate eye; in the case of the human eye, that can be as many as 150 hues.

Can other primates distinguish as many colors as this? That is highly questionable. First, we know that primitive peoples distinguish fewer colors than Westerners. Australian bushmen according to Rivers have three color responses; the first links red, purple and orange; the second, white, yellow and green and the third, black, blue and violet. Nonetheless, some of these people are fine painters. The Japanese have only one word

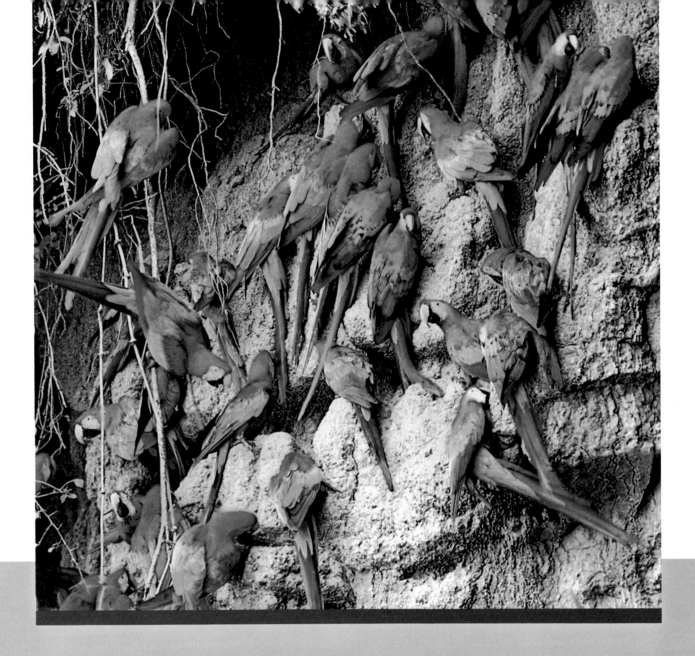

Here we see an example of the color-vision limitations of New World monkeys. The first picture shows normal trichromatic color perception. In the second, there is little perception of reds, and any green is seen as a more neutral shade of white.

for both green and blue, *ao*, even though they can distinguish one from another. Color frequently had a religious as well as a personal meaning for people in ancient societies, but perhaps the capacity to distinguish colors can be explained with an analogy; the Eskimos have nine words for snow while we have only one. It all depends on what you need to see, and by this I mean to be able to identify and set apart. It is possible that other primates have the same visual machinery as we do, but not the same visual memory.

Another opponent system affects the primate color system; this is the brightness/darkness system, the B/D system for short. Both the red/green and the blue/yellow opponent systems function best within the fovea, that small round area of the primate retina most densely packed with cone photoreceptors; the B/D system operates both in the periphery of the eye dominated by rods and the fovea. When rods and cones function at the same time, that is, in medium-light conditions, they share the same neural pathways. As we have discussed in the vision of the cat, the net result of the B/D system is to desaturate color. Colors seen in early morning or at dusk never have the same level of richness as those seen at midday.

Color Vision in Old and New World Monkeys

As is apparent from the wonderful diversity of their faces, all monkeys are not alike. Whether or not those scientists are right in insisting we are more like African apes than other simians, our color vision certainly has more in common with African monkeys such as the macaque than with monkeys of South America. For many New World monkeys, the world is a blue and yellow jungle, and they clamber among white vines and leaves.

The monkeys of Africa and South America result from two separate evolutions, so vast are the physical differences that set them apart, not the least of which are visual. The New World monkeys of South America have prehensile tails, their nostrils are just two holes in the center of their faces, and no New World monkey tested has ever been found to possess normal trichromatic vision. In contrast, the Old World monkeys of Africa lack the prehensile tail, have nostrils that point downward, and all have normal trichromatic vision, including the macaque previously discussed. This is not to say that every type of African primate in captivity has been tested, but of those that have been, for example, baboons, African green monkeys and mandrills, all have had normal trichromatic vision.

The color defect common to all South American monkeys lies in detecting reds. Some of those tested have been dichromats with a total lack of perception of red and green. The New World monkey that has received as much attention from vision scientists as the African macaque is the *Cebus* monkey. Originally all members of this species were thought to be dichromats. But while recent experiments have shown that colors in the longer wavelengths appear less saturated to their eyes and thus are more difficult for them to discriminate, with sufficient training in the laboratory they can learn to distinguish between reds and greens. The squirrel monkey is also deficient in the longer wavelengths, with some deficient in the perception of reds, others in perceiving greens, and still others are just plain dichromats, totally red/green blind. Color blindness is a term rarely used about animals in vision science; these creatures are regarded as simply having an alternate type of visual system.

Color vision is not common in nocturnal creatures, but the *Aotus,* or owl, monkey, another New World monkey, can discriminate colors. Not many colors, mind you. Its vision is poor by human standards, though it has a limited type of trichromatic vision with three different cones. Colors in the short-wavelength area of the spectrum are far more saturated and distinguishable from one another than are the longer-wavelength colors. Above 500nm it requires large differences in wavelengths, as much as 20nm, to discriminate one color from another. But this is far below the rat, which needs at least a 50nm difference. Contrast this with the human eye, which at its most sensitive is able to discriminate changes in wavelength of a single nanometer.

Another monkey that has been singled out for the attention of vision scientists is the tiny marmoset, whose wizened little head holds eyes with limited trichromatic vision, again weak in the longer wavelengths.

Given that the long-wavelength cone was the last to evolve, it should not be surprising that New World monkeys have difficulty in detecting reds. They are in a different stage of evolution and perhaps closer to their nocturnal ancestors than are African or Asian apes.

The Perception of Form

Only the great apes and man show an appreciation for abstract form, though we know that rats prefer mazes with regular patterns and pigeons are able to tell one photograph from another. It is possible that the reason for this lies in an attribute of primate vision that is lacking in most other sub-mammalian creatures and minimal at best in other mammals: stereopsis or three-dimensional depth perception. Here again we see the importance of the neocortex to primate vision. At birth, cells develop in the neocortex of mammals that do nothing but concern themselves with depth and contour. But in order for stereopsis to be truly effective, both hemispheres of the brain must get information from each eye. In more primitive mammals, most visual information is sent to the opposite hemisphere of the brain, but as mammals evolve, the information channeled to the same hemisphere increases, until the split is 50 percent in the primate eye. The activity of the stereoscopic cells in the neocortex is mediated by the mammalian brain's connecting link, the corpus callosum, which coordinates the messages responsible for the convergence of the eyes. Remember that the corpus callosum has an additional function of major importance to visual memory; it suppresses some information so that each hemisphere of the brain stores separate memories and yet provides the link whereby that information can be transferred to the other hemisphere of the brain when needed. Marsupials, without the corpus callosum, must store the same information in both hemispheres, lessening the space available for new memories.

However, creatures are not born with stereopsis, even if they have partial decussation at the optic chiasma. Stereoptic cells develop only with the use of the eyes, and if a mammal is born blind and recovers its sight much later in life, it will never develop stereopsis but, like sub-mammalian creatures, will be forced to use monocular visual clues to guess at distance and depth. A story is told about a man who had been blind from birth and recovered his sight in his forties. After the bandages were removed from his eyes, he was found attempting to climb out of a hospital window. He thought he could put his foot on the ground; he was on the third floor.

For stereopsis to develop a creature must have both partial decussation and the development of the cells in the visual cortex through use of the eyes. Stereoscopic depth perception reaches its apex in the primate eye. Not only is it responsible for our depth vision, but for other qualities of perception that we share with our fellow primates. Lower mammals such as dogs, cats and rabbits must have a flatter image of the world; sub-mammalian creatures, simply a two-dimensional picture. Even the predatory bird with its extraordinary number of photoreceptors, binocular overlap and the magnification of the deep-pitted fovea must depend entirely on what it sees on its visual screen, the two-dimensional retina.

The primate eye has a remarkable sense of texture and detail; we effortlessly distinguish the subtle changes in the tiny patterning of a flower like Queen Anne's lace. We know from behavioral experimentation that the eye of the octopus, the most highly developed invertebrate eye, can distinguish only filled shapes.

Fine acuity is the ability to detect minute changes in contrast across a visual field, to detect an edge or a contour. Earlier, it was pointed out that the finer and more closely packed the photoreceptors, the more precise

and accurate the optical image on the retina. This holds true for the cells of the receptor fields as well. Receptive fields for brightness/darkness function according to the same rules as opponent color fields. A center group of cells responds to the brightness in a particular section of the retina, while those that surround it respond to what is dark. The principle of the center-surround holds, with the information being accepted by the center, inhibited by the surround or vice versa. The finer and more densely packed the cells in the receptive fields, the greater the accuracy of the image projected onto that section of the brain. It is significant that the receptive fields are larger and therefore more crudely responsive in some sections of the brain than in others.

Some receptive fields pass on only color information. Remember that color information vastly improves a creature's vision during daylight; and this information is particularly important to areas of the brain related to the fovea, which is packed with cones. This also should make us more aware of the importance of the fovea. Most of what registers in the visual cortex of the primate is the work of the fovea. The visual areas of the neocortex devoted to the fovea are larger and more numerous.

The form vision of other trichromatic primates should be almost as good as our own despite a more limited range of focal power in the lens. The human child is born with a range of 15 diopters; the monkey or ape has only 10 or 12D.

Simians, like other creatures of the wild, are generally normally or even somewhat farsighted, with the exception of the baboon and mandrill which tend toward nearsightedness, though no apparent reason has been discovered. Since visual attention plays such an important role, an examination of their behavior might re-

veal some clue. We already know, for instance, that domesticated creatures like hens and gerbils tend toward nearsightedness. It would be interesting to find out if there has been any change in the vision of chimps, gorillas or monkeys held in zoos. To my knowledge, no such study has been made.

Pathways to the Brain

The information from the eye is relayed to the brain via the optic nerve and must pass through a way station called the lateral geniculate nucleus, or LGN for short. The LGN also has receptive fields, but these respond less to diffuse light since the center and surround tend to balance one another out and are more sensitive to sharp points of light. (This may be one of the reasons why we get lost in a fog.) The receptive fields of the LGN are comparable to retinal fields in that they do not trigger behavior in the primate.

The LGN path is the most direct path to the brain; from here, visual information is sent on to the visual cortex, the area striata, as it is called from its striped appearance. This region is located at the base of the skull. Its accessories, the inferotemporal or infero-pretemporal areas also have important visual functions, generally in coordination with other faculties.

The entire optic tectum of sub-mammalian species, called the superior colliculus or our reptilian brain, has become only one small part of the mammalian or primate brain. It is considered a more primitive relay station and sends some information on to the brain. It's receptive fields are much larger than those located in the LGN, and therefore its perceptions more limited.

The classical concept of the superior colliculus is as a visuomotor center mediating pupillary responses, eye movements and visual grasping but not the higher processing of perception. But there is a school of thought that now believes it to be more than a way station or second projection area. While the area striata is a more sophisticated analyzer of form, some of its analytical features have apparently been grafted onto the primitive colliculus, though this may not be a part of the conscious mind but instead a crude command station of the unconscious.

There are a variety of theories that attempt to explain how the brain translates vision into perception. These functions are invariably divided into two systems. According to one theory, form analysis is opposed to spatial analysis; in the second theory, one system analyzes foveal information while the other is devoted to peripheral information from the rods; and in the third theory, one system concerns itself with information that comes to the brain from the eye while the other occupies itself with making visual responses. While the jury is still out, the first theory—form analysis operating as one system and spatial analysis as the second system—is considered to be closest to what actually occurs.

What happens when any primate looks at an object in space? First, the eye jumps to localize it. This is known as a saccade. Next, if the object is moving, the eye begins to follow it in a smooth tracking motion designed for recognition. Finally, the eye fixates with a steady gaze and attempts to identify it.

The first jump is monitored by the superior colliculus. Tracking and steady fixation are the work of the LGN. But, as has been pointed out, the eye always makes movements, even during steady fixation. These are called flicks, drifts and tremors and last only about 25 milliseconds.

One part of the brain, probably the superior colliculus, directs the eyes to objects that have been seen before, while another projects scenes that are new back to the brain via the LGN. Lettvin, who has made many studies of the frog eye, believes that even these simple creatures have "sameness" neurons and "newness" neurons.

What we have seen before determines to a large degree what we will look at in the future, which is another way of saying that visual memory interferes with visual attention. Visual memory causes changes in the structure of the protoplasm of the brain called engrams. Once these images become part of our unconscious, they continue to exert an influence over how we, or any primate, will behave, though the memory banks of human beings are significantly larger than those of other primates. We are born with the same size brain as apes, but in the first year or so of our lives, the human neocortex expands dramatically, the soft head of the infant expanding with the neocortex, including the parts of the brain that are devoted to the visual sense.

More than any other organ of sense, vision has released the organism from the bondage of the conditioned reflex. (See R. L. Gregory's *The Intelligent Eye.*) The organism paused to identify an external object, and over the ages its reflections as well as its responses became more numerous and varied as the central nervous system evolved to greater and greater complexity. The intimate connection of eye and brain, the similarity of the nerve cells, the structural mimicry, all point to this conclusion.

The extraordinary adaptability of the eye and its ability to respond in the most varied conditions are without question. One cannot escape the importance of visual attention. Ungulates that spend their lives scanning the horizon for carnivorous predators became horizontally astigmatic by their third year. Domesticated birds become nearsighted though birds are naturally farsighted with, as far as we know, only one wild exception, the flightless kiwi. Primates are farsighted, with the exception of mandrills and human, though some scientists believe that human nearsightedness is cultural, occurring frequently in bookworms. Does the animal need to see at night? Well, that takes a little longer, at least by our standards.

The human retina is the envy of the computer scientist, performing approximately 10 billion calculations every second. While the neurons operate about a million times more slowly than silicon chips, they are capable of doing millions or even billions of operations simultaneously, while the computer operates in a serial, one-step-at-a-time fashion. Since the human eye is so much like the eye of many other primates, there is little reason to doubt that their eyes function almost as well.

The ability to recognize and even prefer certain shapes is widespread in the animal kingdom; for example, poultry prefer circular feed grains, and frogs prefer to escape into openings with parallel horizontal rather than vertical lines, but could the wiring of the eye, or more exactly, its *pre*wiring, predispose us to the recognition of basic shapes to the exclusion of new forms? Or are such forms so implicit in the structure of the universe that we would be less equipped to experience the world visually without their instinctual perception?

Our own vision of the world, which, as Zen poets and language experts like Korzybski remind us, is only a map and not reality, has been extended by devices such as the electron microscope, radar, infrared film, ultraviolet lenses and lights, fiber optics, etc., so that we now have some sense of how the visual maps of other creatures appear to their own eyes. And yet, underlying the flow of images that pass in time and space before the eyes of all creatures is one important physical similarity: Any visual image is nothing more, and certainly nothing less, than varying patterns of light.

Bibliography
Index
Photo Credits

Bibliography

General and Introduction

Burton, Robert. *Animal Senses*. Taplinger Publisher, 1970.

Burtt, E. T. *The Senses of Animals*. London: Wykenham Pub. Ltd., 1974.

Burtt, E. T. *Behavioral Significance of Color*. London: Garland STPM Press, 1969.

Crescitelli, F., ed. "The visual system of vertebrates." *Handbook of Sensory Physiology* Vol. VII/5, Springer-Verlag, 1977.

Droescher, Vitus. *The Magic of the Senses*. E. P. Dutton & Co., 1969.

Duke-Elder, Sir Stuart. *"Systems of opthalmology." The Eye in Evolution,* Vol. I. London: Henry Kimpton, 1958.

Hailman, J. *Optical Signals*. Indiana University Press, 1977.

Lythgoe, J. N. *Ecology of Vision*. Clarendon Press, 1979.

Prince, J. H. *Comparative Anatomy of the Eye*. Springfield (Ill.): Charles C. Thomas, 1956.

Rodiek, R. W. *The Vertebrate Retina*. W. H. Freeman & Co., 1973.

Walls, G. L. *The Vertebrate Eye and Its Adaptive Radiation*. Hafner Publishing Co., 1942.

Wickler, M. *Mimicry in Plants and Animals,* trans. R. D. Martin. London: Weidenfield & Nicholson, 1968.

Forming an Image

Campbell, F. W., and Green, D. G. "Monocular vs. binocular visual acuity." London: *Nature,* Vol. 208, 1965.

Crescitelli, F. W. "The visual cells and visual pigments of the vertebrate eye." *Handbook of Sensory Physiology,* Vol. VII/1, ed. H. J. A. Dartnall. Springer-Verlag, 1972. pp. 245-363.

Daveson, H., ed. "Identity and distribution of visual pigments in the animal world." *The Eye*. London: Academic Press, 1962.

Goldsmith, T. H. "The natural history of invertebrate visual pigments." *Handbook of Sensory Physiology,* Vol. VII/1, ed. H. J. A. Dartnall. Springer-Verlag, 1972.

Mueller, C. G., and Rudolph, M. *Light and Vision*. New York: Time-Life Books, 1968.

Wald, G. "Light and Life." *Scientific American,* October, 1959.

Invertebrates

Autrum, H. J., ed. "Vision in invertebrates—*Invertebrate photoreceptors." Handbook of Sensory Physiology,* Vol. VII/6A. Berlin: Springer-Verlag, 1979.

———. "Vision in invertebrates—invertebrate visual centers and behavior." *Handbook of Sensory Physiology,* Vol. VII/6C, Springer-Verlag, 1981.

Blest, A. D., and Land, M. F. "The physiological optics of Dinopis subrufus L. Koch: A fish lens in a spider." Proceedings. Royal Society B, Vol. 196. pp. 197-222, 1977.

Brues, C. T. "Photographic evidence in the visibility of color patterns to human and insect eye." Proccedings. *American Academy of Arts and Science, Vol. 74, 1941.* pp. 281-5.

Carricaburu, P. "Sous quel aspect les insectes voient-ils les objectes colores." Vision Research 14, 1974. pp. 671-5.

Chapman, R. F. *The Insect's Structure and Function.* Harvard University Press, 1982.

Cousteau, J. Y., and Diole, P. *The Soft Intelligence—Octopus and Squid.* Doubleday, Inc., 1973.

Felix, R. F. Biology of Spiders. Harvard University Press, 1982.

Goldsmith, T. H. "Color vision of insects." *Light and Life,* ed. W. B. McElroy and B. Grass. Johns Hopkins Press, 1961.

Horridge, G. A., ed. *The Compound Eye and Vision of Insects.* Oxford Clarendon Press, 1975.

Kirshfield, K. "The resolution of the lens and compound eyes." *Neural Principles of Vision,* ed. F. Zettler and R. Weiler. Springer-Verlag, 1975.

McCarthy, J. D. *An Introduction to the Behavior of Invertebrates.* George Allen & Unwid Ltd., 1957.

Mazokin-Porschnyakov, G. A. *Insect Vision.* Plenum Press, 1969.

Russell-Hunter, W. D. *A Life of Invertebrates.* Macmillan, 1978.

Swihart, S. L. "A neural basis of color vision in the butterfly, Papilio troilus." *Journal of Insect Phys. 16,* 1970. pp. 1623-36.

———. and Gordon, W. C. "Red receptors in butterflies." London: *Nature,* Vol. 231, 1971. p. 126.

Warner, G. F. *Biology of Crabs.* Van Nostrand and Rheinhold Co., 1977.

Waterman, T. H. *Physiology of Crustacea.* Vol. II. Academic Press, 1961.

Young, J. Z. *The Anatomy and Nervous System of Octopus Vulgaris.* Clarendon Press, 1971.

Fish

Ali, M. A., ed. *Vision in Fish—New Approaches in Research.* Plenum Press, 1974.

Clarke, G. L. "The depth at which fishes see." *Ecology,* Vol. 17, 1936. pp. 452-6.

Harosi, F., and MacNichol, E. F. "Visual pigments of goldfish cones." *Journal of General Physiology,* Vol. 63, 1974. pp. 279-304.

Harvey, E. N. *Bioluminescence.* Academic Press, 1952.

Herring, P. J. "Bioluminescence of marine organisms." London: *Nature,* Vol. 267, 1977. pp. 788-93.

Kinney, J. S., Luria, S. M., and Weitzman, D. O. "Vision of color underwater." *Journal Optical Society of America,* Vol. 57, 1967. pp. 802-9.

McFarland, E. F., and Muntz, F. "Fish with double vision." *Natural History,* Vol. 89, January, 1980. pp. 62-7.

Morland, J. D., and Lythgoe, J. H. "Yellow corneas in fish." *Vision Research,* Vol. 8, 1968. pp. 1377-80.

O'Day, W. T., and Fernandez, H. R. "Aristomias scintillans: a deep-sea fish with visual pigments apparently adapted to its own bioluminescence." *Vision Research,* Vol. 14, 1974. pp. 545-50.

Protasov, V. R. *Vision and Near Orientation of Fish.* Israel Program for Scientific Translation, 1970.

Sosin, M., and Clark, J. *Through a Fish's Eye.* Harper and Row, 1973.

Reptiles and Amphibians

Arden, G. B., and Tansley, K. "The electroretinogram of a diurnal gecko." *Journal of General Physiology,* Vol. 45, 1963. pp. 1145-61.

Barlow, H. B. "Summation and inhibition in the frog's retina." *Journal of General Physiology,* Vol. 119, 1953. pp. 69-88.

Chapman, R. "Spectral sensitivity of the frog in ultraviolet." *Vision Research,* Vol. 14, 1974. pp. 1317-22.

———."Light wavelength and energy preference of the bullfrog: Evidence of color vision." *Journal of Comparative and Physiological Psychology,* Vol. 61, 1966. pp. 429-435.

Eakin, R. *The Third Eye.* University of California Press, 1973.

Fite, K. V., ed. *The Amphibian Visual System.* Academic Press, 1976.

Granda, A. M., and Dvorak, L. A. "Vision in turtles." *Handbook of Sensory Physiology,* Vol. VII/5, ed. F. Crescitelli. Springer-Verlag, 1977.

Harkness, L. "Chameleons use accommodative cues to judge distance." London: *Nature,* Vol. 267, 1977. pp. 346-9.

Hubbard, E. *Eyes and Other Sense Organs of Sea Snakes.* University Park Press, 1975.

Maturana, H. R. Lettvin, J. Y., McCulloch, W. S., and Pitts, W. H. "Anatomy and physiology of vision in the frog (Rana pipiens)." *Journal of General Physiology,* Vol. 43, Suppl. 2, 1960. pp. 129-71.

Newman, E., and Hartline, P. "The infrared vision in snakes." *Scientific American,* March, 1982.

Wall, G. L. "The reptilian retina." *American Journal of Opthalmology,* Vol. 17, 1934. pp. 892-915.

Birds

Bowmaker, J. K. "Color vision in birds and the role of oil droplets." *Trends in Neuroscience,* August, 1980. pp. 196-199.

Fite, K. V. "Anatomical and behavioral correlates of visual acuity in the great horned owl." *Vision Research,* Vol. 13, 1973. pp. 219-230.

Freethy, Ron. *How Birds Work—A Guide to Bird Biology.* Blanford Press, Poole, Dorset, 1982.

Goldsmith, T. H. "Hummingbirds see near ultraviolet light." *Science,* Vol. 207, 1980. pp. 786-788.

Herrenstein, R. J., and Loveland, D. H. "Pigeon perception of letters of the alphabet." *Science,* Vol. 146, 1964. p. 549.

Mathews, G. V. *Bird Navigation.* Cambridge University Press, 1968.

Meyer, D. B. "The avian eye and its adaptation." *Handbook of Sensory Physiology,* Vol. VII/5, ed. F. Crescitelli. Springer-Verlag, 1977.

Milne, L. J., and Milne, M. *Senses of Animals and Men.* Atheneum, 1967.

Simpson, G. G. *Penguins Past and Present.* Yale University Press, 1976.

Snyder, W., and Miller, W. H. "Telephoto lens system of falciform eyes." *Nature,* Vol. 275, 1978. pp. 127-9.

Sturkie, P. D., ed. *Avian Physiology.* Springer-Verlag, 1976.

Young, S. R., and Martin, G. D. "Optics of retinal oil droplets: A model of light collection and polarization in the avian retina." *Vision Research,* Vol. 24, #2, 1984. pp.129-132.

Nocturnal Mammals and Marsupials

Burton, R. *Nature's Nightlife.* Dorset (England): Blanford Press, 1965.

Dominique, P. C. *Ecology and Behavior of Nocturnal Primates and Prosimians in West Africa,* trans. R. D. Martin. New York: Columbia Press, 1977.

Doty, R. W., and Negrao, N. "Forebrain commissures and vision." *Handbook of Sensory Physiology,* Vol. VII/3B, ed. R. Jung. Springer-Verlag, 1973.

Friedman, H. "Color vision in the Virginia opposum." London: *Nature,* Vol. 213, 1967. pp. 835-36.

Griffiths, M. *Biology of Monotremes.* Academic Press, 1958.

Lynn, G. *Marsupials of Australia.* Angus and Robertson, 1967.

Michael, K. M., Fischer, B. E., and Johnson, J. I. "Racoon performance on color discrimination problems." *Journal of Comparative and Physiological Psychology,* Vol. 53, 1960. pp.379-380.

Murphy, C. J., et al. "Visual accommodation in the flying fox." *Vision Research,* Vol. 23, 1983.

Prince, J. *Animals in the Night—Senses After Dark.* Angus and Robertson, 1968.

Stonehouse, B., and Gillmore, D. *Biology of Monotremes.* University Park Press, 1977.

Arden, G. B., and Tansley, K. "Spectral sensitivity of the pure cone retina of the grey squirrel." London: *Journal of Physiology,* Vol. 127, 1955. pp. 592-602.

Autrum, H. J., and Thomas, I. "Comparative physiology of color vision." *Handbook of Sensory Physiology,* Vol. VII/3A, ed. R. Jung. Springer-Verlag, 1973.

Bishop, P. O. "Neurophysiology of binocular single vision and stereopsis." *Handbook of Sensory Physiology,* Vol. VIII, ed. R. Held, et al. Springer-Verlag, 1978.

Cooper, G. F., and Robinson, J.G. "The yellow color of the lenses of the grey squirrel." *Journal of Physiology,* Vol. 203, 1969. pp. 403-410.

Dagge, A., and Foster, J. B. *The Giraffe—Biology and Behavior.* Van Nostrand, 1976.

Darbrowsker, B., Harmata, W., Lenkiewicz, Z., and Wojtusiak, R. J. "Color perception in cows." *Behavioral Process,* Vol. 6, 1981. pp. 1-10.

DeValois, R. L. "Central mechanisms of color vision." *Handbook of Sensory Physiology,* Vol. VII/3A, ed. R. Jung. Springer-Verlag, 1973.

Graham, C. H., ed. *Vision and Visual Perception.* Wiley Publications, 1965.

Hemila, S., Reuter, T., and Virtanen, K. "The evolution of color opponent neurones in color vision." *Vision Research,* Vol. 16, pp. 1359-62.

Hobson, E. S. "Orientation and feeding in sea lions. London: *Nature,* Vol. 210, 1966. p. 326.

Huebel, D. H. "Integrative processes in central visual pathways of the cat." *Information Processing Approaches to Visual Perception,* ed. Ralph Habor. Holt, Rinehart & Winston, 1969.

Hughes, Austin. "The topography of vision in mammals of contrasting lifestyle." *Handbook of Sensory Physiology,* Vol. VII/5, ed. F. Crescittelli. Springer-Verlag, 1977.

Jacobs, G. A., *Comparative Color Vision.* Academic Press, 1981.

Martin, R. J. *Mammals of the Ocean.* G. P. Putnam, 1977.

Nuboer, J. W. F. "Spectral discrimination in a rabbit." *Documentat Opthalmologica,* Vol. 30, 1971. pp. 279-298.

Prince, J. *The Rabbit in Eye Research.* Springfield, (Ill): Charles C. Thomas, 1964.

Rosengren, A. "Experiments in color discrimination in dogs." *Acta Zoologica Fennica,* Vol. 121, 1969. pp. 3-19.

Tribe, D. E., and Gordon, J. G. "The importance of color vision to the grazing sheep." *Journal of Agricultural Science,* Vol. 39, 1950. pp. 313-315.

Blakeslee, B., and Jacobs, G. H. *The Squirrel Monkey. Folia Primatologica,* 1981.

Bowmaker, J. K., Dartnall, H. J., and Mollen, J. D. "The violet sensitive receptors of primate retinas." *Investigative Opthamology and Vision Science Supplement,* Vol. 18, 1979. p.31.

———, Dartnall, H. J., et al. "The visual pigments of rods and cones in the rhesus monkey Macca mulatta." London: *Journal of Physiology,* Vol. 274, 1978. pp.329-48.

Boynton, R. J. *Human Color Vision.* Holt, Rinehart & Winston, 1979.

Gregory, R. L. *Eye and Brain.* Macmillan, 1966.

———. *The Intelligent Eye.* Macmillan, 1970.

Gross, C. G. "Visual perception and neurophysiology—receptive fields of the inferotemporal cortex in monkeys." *Handbook of Sensory Physiology,* Vol. VII/3B, ed. R. Jung. Springer-Verlag, 1973.

Hochberg, J. E. *Perception.* Prentice Hall, Inc., 1964.

Jung, R. "Visual perception and neurophysiology. *Handbook of Sensory Physiology,* Vol. VII/3A, ed. R. Jung. Springer-Verlag, 1973.

Kandell, E. R., and Schwartz, J. H. *Principles of Neural Science.* Elsevier, 1981.

MacKay, D. M. "Visual stability and voluntary eye movements." *Handbook of Sensory Physiology,* Vol. VII/3A, ed. R. Jung. Springer-Verlag, 1973.

Motokawa, K. *Physiology of Color and Pattern Vision.* Igaku Shoin Ltd., 1970.

Oyama, T., Furusalea, T., and Kito, T. "Color vision in men and animals." *Scientific American,* December, 1979.

Pilbeam, D. "The descent of hominoids and hominids." *Scientific American,* March, 1984.

Sprague, J. M., Berlucchi, G., and Rizzolati, G. "The role of the superior colliculus and pretectum in vision." *Handbook of Sensory Physiology,* Vol. VII/3B, ed. R. Jung. Springer-Verlag, 1973.

Stephenson, P. H. "The evolution of color vision in primates." *Journal of Human Evolution,* Vol. 2, 1973. pp. 379-384.

Stone, J., and Freeman, R. B., Jr. "Neurophysiology of form discrimination." *Handbook of Sensory Physiology,* Vol. VII/3A, ed. R. Jung. Springer-Verlag, 1973.

Index

A

Ablepharus 81
Adelie 96
Agnatha 51
Alevin 67
Alligator 75, 79
Amberjack 59
Amblyopsid 62
Amia 51, 54
Amphibians 51, 60, 68-74, 76, 103, 106, 116
Anabas fish 51
Anableps 50
Anemone 34
Angwantibo 111
Anolis 81
Antelope 104
Ants 23
Anurans 69
Apes 127, 132
Apus apus 96
Arachnids 14
Archerfish 53, 93
Architeuthis 9, 48
Aristomias 63
Arthropoda 14
Auks 94
Axolotl 69

B

Baboon 132, 133
Badger 109
Bat 106-108
Bathythannia 48
Beaver 115
Bees xiii, xviii, 8, 13, 21, 23, 26, 27, 29,
   32-33, 37, 73, 92, 106
Beetles xi, 21, 36
Bird snake 87
Birds xiii, xviii, 3, 15, 18, 20, 30, 76, 77-78,
   79, 88-100, 103, 113, 116, 134
Bittern 100
Boa constrictor xi, 84, 85
Boid 83
Bowfin 51
Boxfish 58
Bush babies 110-111
Butterflies 18, 23, 24, 27, 29, 31, 32, 33, 37
Butterfly fish 52, 58

C

Cat 6, 31, 103, 104, 116-118, 124, 133
Caterpillar 1
Catfish 49, 62
Cave fish 9
Cephalopod 9, 13, 19, 42, 43-48, 53, 92
Ceratoid angler fish 62
Cetaceans 124
Chameleon 80-81
Cheetah 118
Chelonia mydas 77
Chelonians 75, 77, 80
Chickens xv, 1, 90, 99, 113

Chimaera shark 62
Chimpanzee 127, 133, 136, 139
Chondrosteans 51
Cilium 13
Clemmys insculpta 77
Cobra 85
Cockatoo 115
Cockroach 36
Coelacanth 23, 50
Cone shell 11
Copelia xiii, 1, 39
Copperhead 84
Coral 10
Cormorant 94, 96
Crab 39
Crab spider 18, 20
Crayfish 39
Cricket 28, 111
Crocodile 75, 79-80, 83, 87, 103
Crossopterygian 69
Crusatceans 1, 9, 14, 39-43, 53
Cuttlefish 47
Cyprinidae 65

D

Daddy longlegs 18
Damselflies 26, 28
Deer 123-124
Dinosaurs 75, 125
Dipnoi 51
Dipoans 69
Diprodont 106
Dog 115, 119, 136
Dogfish shark 31
Dolphins 95, 101, 124, 125
Doodlebug 14
Douricouli monkey 103
Dragonfish 64
Dragonflies 1, 23, 28, 30, 32, 36
Dryophis 87
Duck 94
Dugong 124, 136

E

Eagle 88, 93
Earthworm 9, 10
Eel 49, 67, 79
Elasmobranch 50-51, 60
Elephant 123

F

Falcon 88, 93
Fiddler crab 40
Fireflies xii
Fish xi, 6, 8, 9, 18, 33, 49-67, 69, 76, 78,
   104, 113, 115, 116, 125
Fishing bat 108
Flashlight fish 63
Flies 14, 21-25, 26, 28, 30
Flounder 50
Flour moth 26
Frog xvii, 69, 73-74, 78

Frond worm 11
Fruit bat 105, 108

G

Gar 51, 54
Gecko 80, 124
Gerbil 133
Giant squid 48
Gibbon 127
Giraffe 123
Glass snake 80
Goldfish 65, 118
Gopherus polyphemus 77
Gorilla 127, 128, 133
Green monkey 132
Grimaldi teuthis 48
Guinea pig 113
Gull 94, 95
Gulper eel 62
Guppy 66

H

Halibut 57
Hammerhead shark 50, 61
Hare 104
Harlequin 58
Hatchetfish 63
Hawk xiii, 88, 89, 90, 93
Hen 133
Hippopotami 104, 123
Histioteuthis 48
Holosteans 51, 69
Horse 122
Horseshoe crab xvii, 9, 42
Housefly 32
Hover fly 31
Hummingbird 90, 97-98

I

Idiacanthus 50
Iguana 80
Insects xi, 1, 3, 9, 14, 21-39, 45, 76, 115
Ipnops 62

J

Jawless fish 1
Jellyfish 9, 10, 48

K

Kangaroo 106
King crab 42
Kingfisher 93-94
Kiwi 88, 99, 134
Krill 88, 99, 134

L

Lacertilians 75
Lamprey 51, 87
Lemon shark 61
Lemur 104, 110, 127
Leopard 50

Limilus 9
Lion 14, 50
Lizards xi, 15, 75-76, 80-83, 87
Lobster 24, 39, 41, 103
Loon 94
Lorisines 111
Lungfish 51, 69

M

Macaque monkey 8, 132
Mammals 112-126
Manatee 126, 134
Mandrill 132, 133, 134
Manta 50, 60
Marlin 59
Marmoset 132
Mice 87, 122
Mollusks 10, 11, 13
Monkey xv, 138, 143-145
Monotremes 113
Mosquitoes 26
Moth 27, 32, 36, 103, 108
Mudskipper 51, 68

N

Nassau grouper 58
Nautilus 11
Newt 76, 78, 79, 81, 82
Nightingale 107

O

Octopi 9, 43, 47, 133
Ophidians 75-76
Opossum 106
Orangutan 127
Ostrich 88
Otter 115
Owl xiii, 62, 96, 101
Owl monkey 132

P

Pachystomias 63
Parrot 90
Penguin 96
Perch 52, 59, 115
Pigeon 78, 90, 99, 116, 132
Pike 59
Pinnipedia 124
Pit viper xi, 83, 84
Placoderm 50
Plankton 48, 52, 55, 94
Potto 111
Poultry 134
Prairie dog 77, 119-121
Praying mantis 15, 36
Promisians 110-111
Protocornus 63
Protozoa 13
Pseudemys 77
Pygidiid 62
Python 84

R

Rabbit 104, 113, 114, 115, 118-119, 132, 133
Raccoon 109
Rat 116, 122
Rattlesnake 84
Rays 50, 60
Razorbill 94
Reptiles 75-87, 103
Rhynchocephalia 75, 87
Rodents 110

S

Saber-toothed tiger 115
Salamander 69, 71, 72, 73
Salmon 50, 67
Sandalops 48
Scallop 11, 13, 17
Scorpion 14, 39
Sea anemones 10
Sea snake 79-80
Sea turtle 77, 79
Sea urchin 10
Seal 9, 80, 87, 124, 125
Shag 94
Shark 13, 49, 50, 52, 56, 60, 61
Shearwater 94
Sheep 134
Shrew 111
Shrike 88
Shrimp 39
Siamese cat 117
Sirenians 124
Skink 80, 81
Skunk 109
Slowworm 80
Snakes 75-76, 83-87, 113
Snipe 100
Sole 57
Sparrow 89
Sphenodon 75
Spider shell 11
Spiders 9, 14-20, 39, 106
Sponge 9
Squid 9, 47, 125
Squirrel 77, 109, 119-121
Stallions 115
Starfish 9, 10
Sturgeon 44, 50-51, 55, 56, 113

T

Tadpole 69, 87
Tarsier 101, 110
Tasmanian devil 106, 116
Terns 95
Terrapins 75-76, 77
Thelotornis kirklandi 87
Toad 69-70, 73-74, 78, 106
Tortoise 75-76, 77
Tree shrew 127
Tree snake 87
Trilobite 9
Trout 59
Tuatara lizard 87
Tuna 94
Tupaia glis 111, 127
Turbot 57
Turtles 75-76, 77-79, 83, 113

U

Ungulates 103, 122-123
Urodeles 69, 71

W

Wallaby 106
Walrus 124
Warblers 96
Wasp 15, 73
Water moccasin 84
Western lizard 87
Whale 13, 43, 48, 103, 124-126
White wagtail 90
Wolf spider 16
Woodpecker 90

Y

Yellow tang 52

Z

Zebra 122-123

Photo Credits

Neil G. McDaniel/Tom Stack & Associates
Leonard Lee Rue III/Bruce Coleman, Inc.
Tom Stack/Tom Stack & Associates
George D. Dodge/Bruce Coleman, Inc.
Kjell B. Sandved/Bruce Coleman, Inc.
Chris Newbert/Bruce Coleman, Inc.
Curtis Williams/Natural Science Photos
Sue Drafahl
Chris Newbert/Bruce Coleman, Inc.
Robert P. Carr/Bruce Coleman, Inc.
J. Fennell/Bruce Coleman, Inc.
Robert L. Dunne/Bruce Coleman, Inc.
Jack Drafahl
Dwight R. Kuhn/Bruce Coleman, Inc.
Tom Stack/Tom Stack & Associates
Jack Drafahl
Jack Drafahl
Jack Drafahl
Jack Drafahl
Kim Taylor/Bruce Coleman, Inc.
L. West
Mike Price/Bruce Coleman, Inc.
Mantis Wildlife Films
Dwight R. Kuhn/Bruce Coleman, Inc.
Jane Burton/Bruce Coleman, Inc.
S. L. Craig, Jr./Bruce Coleman, Inc.
E. R. Degginger/Bruce Coleman, Inc.
Dwight R. Kuhn/Bruce Coleman, Inc.
George D. Dodge/Bruce Coleman, Inc.
David Scharf
David Scharf
Peter Ward/Bruce Coleman, Inc.
Terry Domico/Earth Images
Terry Domico/Earth Images
Kjell B. Sandved/Bruce Coleman, Inc.
E. R. Degginger/Bruce Coleman, Inc.
E. R. Degginger/Bruce Coleman, Inc.
P. A. Hinchliffe/Bruce Coleman, Inc.
John Akester/Bruce Coleman, Inc.
Connie Shaw/Bruce Coleman, Inc.
Sue Drafahl
Walter Deas/Seaphot
Jane Burton/Bruce Coleman, Inc.
Jack Drafahl
Jack Drafahl
Jane Burton/Bruce Coleman, Inc.
Jack Drafahl
James M. Cribb/Bruce Coleman, Inc.

William H. Amos/Bruce Coleman, Inc.
Barry E. Parker/Bruce Coleman, Inc.
Anne Wertheim/Bruce Coleman, Inc.
Ron and Valerie Taylor/Bruce Coleman, Inc.
Tropical Fish Hobbyist
M. Timothy O'Keefe
Dwight R. Kuhn/Bruce Coleman, Inc.
Hans Reinhard/Bruce Coleman, Inc.
M. Timothy O'Keefe
Jack Drafahl
Chris Newbert/Bruce Coleman, Inc.
R. L. Sefton/Bruce Coleman, Inc.
Chris Newbert/Bruce Coleman, Inc.
E. R. Degginger/Bruce Coleman, Inc.
E. R. Degginger/Bruce Coleman, Inc.
Warren Williams/Seaphot
George Marler/Bruce Coleman, Inc.
George Marler/Bruce Coleman, Inc.
William H. Amos/Bruce Coleman, Inc.
Herve Chaumeton/Bassot-Nature
Herve Chaumeton/Bassot-Nature
Ken Lucas/Seaphot
G. E. Schmida/Bruce Coleman, Inc.
Hans Reinhard/Bruce Coleman, Inc.
Hans Reinhard/Bruce Coleman, Inc.
Dan Wells
Jeff Foott/Bruce Coleman, Inc.
Alan Blank/Bruce Coleman, Inc.
C. Mattison/Natural Science Photos
G. E. Schmida/Bruce Coleman, Inc.
Jane Burton/Bruce Coleman, Inc.
Michael Fogden/Bruce Coleman, Inc.
Michael Fogden/Bruce Coleman, Inc.
Dwight R. Kuhn/Bruce Coleman, Inc.
Dwight R. Kuhn/Bruce Coleman, Inc.
Robert Abrams/Bruce Coleman, Inc.
Robert Abrams/Bruce Coleman, Inc.
J. C. Carton/Bruce Coleman, Inc.
E. R. Degginger/Bruce Coleman, Inc.
Kim Taylor/Bruce Coleman, Inc.
E. R. Degginger/Bruce Coleman, Inc.
S. L. Craig, Jr.
S. L. Craig, Jr./AGA Corporation
Lynn M. Stone/Bruce Coleman, Inc.
Alan Blank/Bruce Coleman, Inc.
George D. Dodge and D. R. Thompson/Bruce Coleman, Inc.
Norman Tomalin/Bruce Coleman, Inc.
Laura Riley/Bruce Coleman, Inc.

Cameron Davidson/Bruce Coleman, Inc.
Cameron Davidson/Bruce Coleman, Inc.
E. R. Degginger/Bruce Coleman, Inc.
R. Kemp/Natural Science Photos
Jen and Des Bartlett/Bruce Coleman, Inc.
J. C. Carton/Bruce Coleman, Inc.
Bob and Clara Calhoun/Bruce Coleman, Inc.
M. Konishi
Fred J. Alsop III/Bruce Coleman, Inc.
James H. Carmichael/Bruce Coleman, Inc.
S. C. Bisserot
Sandra Sinclair
Sandra Sinclair
Jane Burton/Bruce Coleman, Inc.
Michael Fogden/Bruce Coleman, Inc.
Gary Milburn/Tom Stack & Associates
Rod Williams/Bruce Coleman, Inc.
Carol Hughes/Bruce Coleman, Inc.
Jane Burton/Bruce Coleman, Inc.
S. L. Craig/Bruce Coleman, Inc.
K. Ammann/Bruce Coleman, Inc.
Gary R. Zahm/Bruce Coleman, Inc.
S. L. Craig, Jr.
Wendell Metzen/Bruce Coleman, Inc.
Wendell Metzen/Bruce Coleman, Inc./retouching by M. Meloy
Kjell B. Sandved/Bruce Coleman, Inc.
Leonard Lee Rue III/Bruce Coleman, Inc.
Len Rue, Jr./Bruce Coleman, Inc.
Len Rue, Jr./Bruce Coleman, Inc.
James Hudnall and Leigh Wilks/Seaphot
Tony Arruza/Bruce Coleman, Inc.
Tony Arruza/Bruce Coleman, Inc.
Dotte Larsen/Bruce Coleman, Inc.
Larry Aumiller/Bruce Coleman, Inc.
Steve Solum/Bruce Coleman, Inc.
Kenneth W. Fink/Bruce Coleman, Inc.
David Overcash/Bruce Coleman, Inc.
Gunter Zeisler
Gunter Zeisler/retouching by M. Meloy

Illustrations by Ann Jasperson

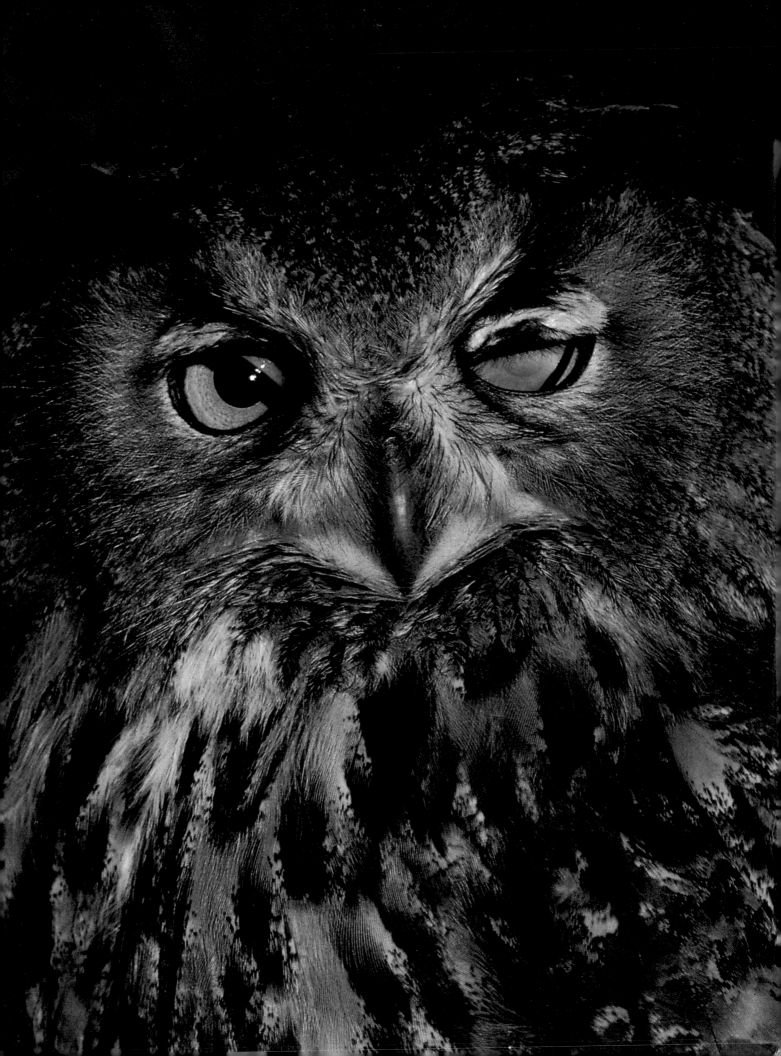